Not in Kansas Anymore

A Memoir of the Farm, New York City, and Life with ALS

Robert E. Paulson

Dedication

This book is for my wife, Maureen, the best part of every day, and for my sons, Joshua, Luke and James (Jake), all of whom encouraged me to write down the stories I had told them over the years about growing up on a farm, making my way east, and finally coming to New York.

I thank you for your steadfast love, support and patience throughout our lives together, and particularly during the past twelve years, as you have helped me cope in the best possible way with the ALS disease.

I dedicate this book to all of you.

Acknowledgements

For a long and pleasurable career in patent law, I owe a debt of gratitude to the mentorship of many fine attorneys. I started my career under the tutorship of Hobart Durham, Granville Pine and Warren Rotert, learned still more from Jack Foley and John Vassil in mid-career, and was privileged to work most closely with John Diaz, a particularly talented and dedicated patent lawyer, over the last some 20 or more years. We never exchanged sharp words, and the credo was simple: Always do the very best you can for each and every client, large or small.

In recent years, I have been very grateful for the assistance of a new group of associates—each and every one of the caregivers who have so faithfully attended to all my wishes and needs and who have helped me with tasks I can no longer do for myself. Thanks to them all. I want to mention Doctor Abdel Zerzif, a medical student with a knack for tying neckties; Oliver Pua, who filled the roles of personal attendant, paralegal and part-time secretary for nine years; Jose Molina, who has been with me since the beginning and remains my "numero uno" companion; Karen Jack, a special nurse/respiratory therapist, who brings smiles and laughter to her work; Grace Kozak, who always gives me extra time at the end of her shift; Peter Fernezy, who gives up his weekends so that I am up and in my wheelchair every day of the week; and John Nelson, a superb massage/physical therapist who has kept me limber for more than 10 years while I have been confined to my wheelchair.

For their dedication and competence, I want to thank the doctors who have successfully shepherded me through the complications of the ALS disease over the past 12 years and also the many outstanding members of the medical support staffs at their respective hospitals. They include Dr. Lewis Rowland at New York Presbyterian; the unnamed paramedic who revived me from a respiratory failure with an emergency intubation and brought me to Mass General; Dr. Inocencia Carrano at Helen Hayes Hospital; and Dr. Louis DePalo, Dr. Diane Duffy, Dr. Dale Lange and Dr. Daniel J. Krellenstein at Mt. Sinai.

I also want to express my deep appreciation to all our friends, our family, Pastor John Smucker and his wife Irene, my law partners, and the business associates who have so generously contributed their time and financial support for the benefit of my home healthcare fund over the past several years. Your dedication and loyalty have allowed me to enjoy a slice of life that otherwise would not have been possible.

I also owe special thanks to a series of people who made my stories appear in the form of a beautiful book: my niece, Lara Kroeker, who created the book cover; Gwendolyn Penner, who designed the layout of the book; Sarah Yates of Gemma B. Publishing c.o.b. Gemma B. Inc., who deftly handled the details of publishing; Gail Furgal, who thought of the very apt title for the book; and Eric Chan and Heather Schatz, who took the photograph that appears on the back cover that shows me writing on my computer, using only my eyes. And for the eye-controlled computer, I thank Debra Zeitlin at the Helen Hayes Hospital in West Haverstraw, New York, and Jim Stuart at Eye Response Technologies, Inc., Charlottesville, Virginia.

Finally, I must thank Dale R. Burg for her valuable editing and organizing insights and for prodding me to recall more information than I ever imagined was stored away in my head. Dale has been a dear family friend for more than 20 years. A visit with her is always uplifting, as she never fails to have a funny story to tell.

Contents

Part Two: In the City

Part Three: Living with ALS

Postscripts

Tempora mutantur, nos et mutamur in iltis.
Times change, and we change with them.

My very lucky life

My streak of good luck began even before I was born. In 1912, the young woman who would become my mother postponed her plans to sail to New York on the new ship Titanic.

I was lucky to be born!

What's more, I was lucky to be born in my mother's bedroom on a farm in the middle of Kansas. I enjoyed many boyhood pleasures—fishing in hidden creeks, walking barefoot in the mud after a summer rain, and squirting warm milk from a cow's teat across the barn floor into the mouth of a cat sitting on his hind legs. My favorite pastime was to curl up in a warm pile of straw with my pigs on a wintry afternoon.

I was lucky to spend my first five school years in a one-room schoolhouse. Being taught at one level while being exposed to lessons several levels higher is an educational experience I would recommend to anyone.

I was lucky to live near a small town settled by Swedish immigrants that offered a fine arts college and a rich history in music appreciation. While still a boy soprano at the age of fifteen, I was lucky to perform the title role in a college production of *Amahl and the Night Visitors,* which led me to enjoy a lifelong hobby of singing.

I was lucky to be able to study nuclear engineering at Kansas State University and thereafter make my way east to work days at the Atomic Energy Commission and attend night law school at Georgetown University in Washington D.C.

I was lucky to join the Morgan & Finnegan law firm in 1963 as the result of a chance meeting with a classmate at Georgetown. I flourished there as a patent attorney and thoroughly enjoyed a 40-year career.

I was extraordinarily lucky to father three lanky and tall, bright, handsome and devoted sons—Josh, Luke and Jake—each of whom has been a source of much love and cause for pride. Josh, a graduate of Hamilton College, is married to Tammy Janulis and works in finance/investment management. Luke, who holds a degree in geology, recently graduated from the New York Police Academy, and as a hobby he plays drums with a rock band. Jake has been working part-time while composing and producing music for his rap group, "Team Facelift," and pursuing a career in emergency medical services with the New York Fire Department.

The greatest stroke of luck, though, was to have met Maureen Dowling, the love of my life, and to have had her agree to marry me. A graduate of St. Johns University in New York, she taught elementary school in the suburb of White Plains for ten years before becoming a full-time mother. For the past few years, she has been a volunteer instructor in early childhood development (assisting mothers of children aged three months to three years), and she has taught English to young Spanish mothers at a social service agency.

"For better or for worse, in sickness and in health." Following those marriage vows to the letter, Maureen has steadfastly and courageously stood by me for 39 years. No one could ask for a more devoted and loving partner.

When I was about 56 or 57, my life took a dramatic turn. I experienced the onset of what I would eventually learn was ALS (amyotrophic lateral sclerosis), commonly known as Lou Gehrig's Disease.

ALS is a strange and rare affliction. It begins with a slow deterioration of the muscles in the arms, hands and legs. Ultimately, they no longer function. Over time, the involuntary muscles that control breathing are also affected. The patient will eventually die unless doctors perform a tracheostomy and a mechanical ventilator takes over the life-sustaining task of forcing air into and out of the lungs. There are only about 5,000 cases of ALS diagnosed per year in all of the United States, and scientists do not yet know if its cause is environmental or hereditary.

The first signs of my ALS showed up slowly and subtly in the spring and summer of 1993, when I experienced unusual fatigue in my leg and stomach muscles.

By 1996, my ALS had been diagnosed, and by 1998, I was confined to a wheelchair. Still, I was able to continue practicing law until June 2003, when my disability forced me to retire. Less than six months later, on a trip to Boston in early December, I suffered a respiratory failure. I woke up in the ICU of Massachusetts General Hospital, with a tracheostomy, a stomach feeding tube and a life support ventilator. I spent three weeks there recovering.

In January 2004, after an additional three-week stay in a rehabilitation facility where my family, my caretakers and I learned to manage my new equipment and regimen, I was lucky to have a second chance to live. As I write this with my eye-controlled computer, I'm in the fifth year of my new life.

Though I have no function in my limbs, I continue to feel good. I have no loss of sensory perception, nor has my brain function been affected. I can breathe comfortably thanks to the amazing technical sophistication, reliability and portability of a state-of-the-art mechanical ventilator. It is set to help me take in the appropriate volume of air and to breathe at a normal rate. But it is sensitive enough to add volume or frequency in response to my attempts to breathe in unusual circumstances: for example, when the hose has been briefly disconnected while I am moved from the wheelchair to the bed, when I am anxious, or when there is fluid buildup in my lungs.

Still, living with ALS in the later stages of the disease is difficult and frustrating. At this point, I can no longer use the muscles controlling my vocal cords, lower jaw and tongue, so speech is virtually impossible. Since I am unable to speak, gesture or point, my attempts to communicate are arduous and slow, and I am virtually locked in an inanimate body. Such an existence can be a lonely one.

Fortunately, at about the same time as my voice production weakened so that I could manage only a word or two between gasps for breath, I was given a voice-production computer that is controlled by a camera trained on my eye. As my eye scans a keyboard on the lower half of the computer screen, the computer types my words and speaks them aloud. The computer allows me to communicate all my thoughts, questions and needs in every detail and nuance. In one respect, I have an edge over oral speech, since there is a written record of all that I say.

Maureen and my family have insisted on keeping me at home. With their help and that of caregivers, I continue to live comfortably in the Upper East Side apartment building in New York City where my children grew up. I am out and about almost every day, not only to the nearby parks but also to movies, cafes, concerts and museums—even, on occasion, to the opera, ballet or a Broadway show.

Though managing this situation has been financially difficult, our family and friends have continued to rally together in order to support my being cared for at home. For that, I am so very lucky.

I had a childhood very unlike those of my sons, who were born and raised in New York City. Like Dorothy voyaging to Oz, I too left Kansas and the farm behind and found myself on an exciting and surprising journey, one which took a totally unpredictable course when I became afflicted with ALS.

I began this memoir for my children and any others who might enjoy my recollections of growing up as a farm boy, going to school and beginning my career almost fifty years ago, then enjoying a challenging and rewarding life as a patent lawyer and family man in New York City. Ultimately, I decided to include some of the details of living with ALS as well, in the hope that others similarly affected might find something of interest and perhaps of benefit in reading about my experiences.

ALS has stolen many of my physical abilities, but, thanks to modern technology, it has not stolen my ability to live—which is, at its core, the ability to understand, enjoy and communicate. All of these, I can do.

We've all heard the phrase "Life isn't fair," and some say the phrase applies to me. Believe me, I've had that thought myself many times. But upon reflection, I know of no one who has been luckier in life than I. I hope, after you read the pages that follow, you will agree.

Part One: On the Farm

PROLOGUE

A strange twist of fate determined that I would exist. My mother, Ellen Amalia Elisabet Karlsson, born in 1893, immigrated from Landskrona, Sweden to America in 1908. From Ellis Island, she made her way to Chicago, where a cousin was living. There, she found household work with a large family for a number of years.

In early 1912, she made a family visit back to Sweden. For her return to the United States, she bought a ticket to sail on the Titanic, a new and glamorous ocean liner about to make its much-heralded maiden voyage across the Atlantic from Southampton, England to New York. However, a family member was to be married a few days after the scheduled departure. At the last minute, my mother decided to stay for the wedding and exchanged her ticket for a later passage.

Everyone knows the story of how the "unsinkable" Titanic struck an iceberg and went down on April 15, 1912 en route off the coast of Newfoundland. Nearly 1500 passengers perished in that terrible accident. Mother always said she very likely would not have been among the survivors, as she could afford passage only in one of the rooms on the lower levels, where the most

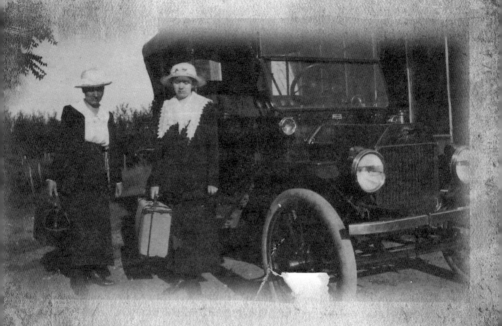

My mother's first cousins,
Ellen and Lillian Malmstrom,
visit the Paulson farm (c1912)

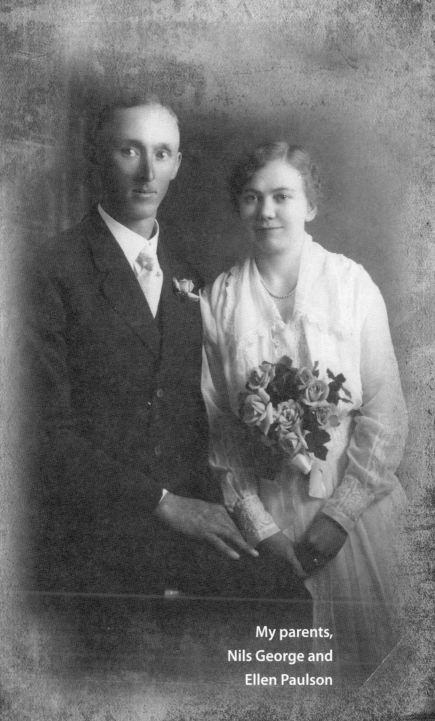

My parents,
Nils George and
Ellen Paulson

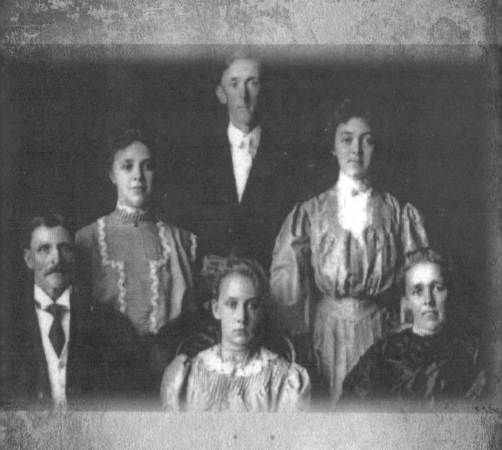

My father, Nils George (back row); my grandparents, John and Elisabet Paulson (center); my aunts, Helga Paulson Jacobson Oberholser, Signe Paulson Anderson and Agnes Paulson Hillgren (c1914)

fatalities occurred.

But for my mother's change of mind, this story would not have been written.

Having returned safely to America, she then traveled to San Francisco to do household work with another family. On her way west, she stopped off in Topeka, Kansas to visit her cousins, Ellen and Lillian Malmstrom. The three of them paid a visit to the Paulson family in Lindsborg, about a three-hour drive from Topeka, and that's where she met Nils George Paulson, my father.

She remained in contact by mail with George, as he was called, over the next five years. By the time World War I ended in 1918—she often recalled how people embraced and danced in the streets in celebration—her long correspondence with George had blossomed into a romance, and he proposed to her by letter. Shortly thereafter, she traveled back to the Paulson family home, where the couple was married on November 5, 1919.

The 320-acre farm where they lived had been purchased by my grandparents, Jons (John) Peter and Elisabet (Pettersson) Paulson, who immigrated to that part of the United States from Sweden in the early 1880s. It was near the center of a large, fertile land area in central Kansas known as the Smoky Valley and four miles southeast of the town of Lindsborg.

Bordered by the Smoky Hill River, the town was settled by Swedish immigrants in about 1868. Since the founding of Bethany College in 1881, Lindsborg has been a center of Kansas religious, cultural and artistic activity. It is home to annual renditions of Handel's *Messiah* and Bach's *Passion According to St. Matthew*, performed by a 300-member chorus made up of local farm and townspeople, the college orchestra and guest

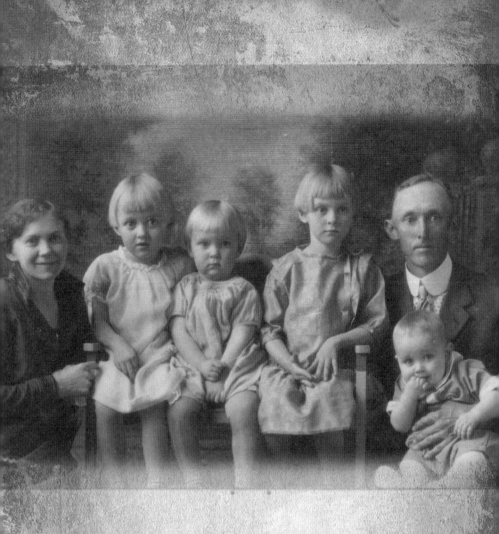

From left, Mother, sisters
Ruth, Eleanor, Georgette,
Father and brother Paul
(December 1926)

solo artists. The bi-annual *Svensk Hyllningsfest* October festival celebrates the town's Scandinavian roots with a parade, folk dancing, and the naming of a queen, the oldest living woman of Swedish descent in the community. The Sandzen Memorial Art Gallery houses works by the renowned French artist Birger Sandzen, who was a professor of art at the college. Not least of all, the town is celebrated as the home of the "Terrible Swedes," the college football team of 1902-03 that defeated such rivals as Oklahoma University. Today Lindsborg remains a farming community of about 3,000 people, most of Swedish ancestry.

In 1887, my father was born on the family farm, as were his sisters, Agnes, Signe and Helga. So were my siblings and I. On June 27, 1937, I became the seventh and last child to be delivered in my mother's bedroom. She was then 43 and my father was 50. My sisters Georgette, Ruth and Eleanor were 16, 14 and 12, respectively, and my brothers Paul, John, Richard and Arnold were 11, 7 and 4.

I have no recollection of my father, who died of stomach cancer nineteen months after my birth. Until her own death 42 years later, my mother remained on the farm.

LOSS

At the time of my birth, life was going well for the Paulsons of Lindsborg. In 1927, their farming efforts had been successful enough so that my parents were able to take a three-week vacation back to Sweden, taking along their four children aged 6 and under, Georgette, Eleanor, Ruth and Paul.

The Great Depression of the early 1930s, which brought much suffering to the country as a whole, had only a slight

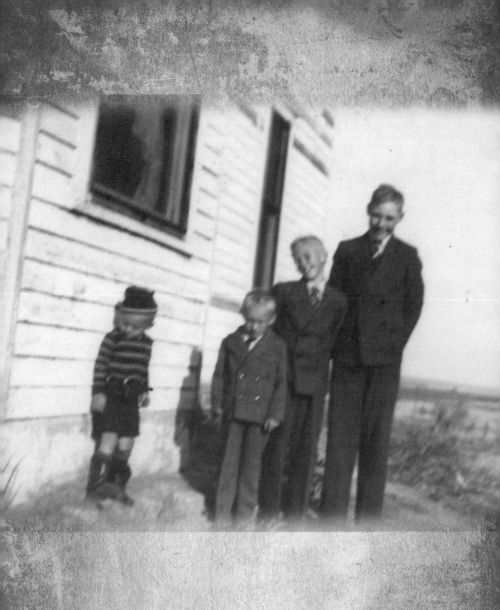

Me, age 3, and my
brothers, aged 7,
10 and 14 (1941)

impact on our family. Even with very little money, a farmer can live quite well off his land, growing every vegetable under the sun and raising his own chickens, cows, and pigs.

To expand the original 320 acres of the farm, my grandfather, relying on my father's help with the farm work, had purchased an additional 80-acre tract of cropland and another 320 acres of pastureland for cattle grazing. In 1938, with 720 acres, my father was poised to take full advantage of the country's booming need for food products in support of the oncoming war effort. Mom often showed me a receipt from that year showing that my father had sold several head of cattle for $4,000. In those days, that was big money, and it was indicative of what the future might have been for our family. There is no telling how my father would have prospered and expanded, particularly with four young boys in the pipeline to help with the farm work.

But his death the following year doomed those possibilities. The loss was surely devastating to my mother, but she revealed it to me on only two occasions that I recall.

On a side of the front yard of our house opposite the driveway, there was a plot about 12 feet square, enclosed with chicken wire—an all-purpose thin fencing wire with openings about an inch wide. For as long as I could remember, it contained mostly weeds. One day I asked Mom why there was a fence around a weed patch. "Oh, Bobby," she said sadly, "that used to be my flower garden. I just lost interest after your father died."

On another occasion, I realized that although I had sat beside her for years during church services after Sunday school and joined in lustily for the hymn singing, Mom never sang along with the rest of us. I asked her why.

"I used to sing. I loved singing," she said. "But when your father died, I lost my voice."

My mother was a small person, only 5'3", while my father was a towering 6'4"—when the average man his age was only about 5'6". He must truly have been a larger-than-life presence to her.

RESPONSIBILITIES

The loss of our father had an immediate effect on our family.

Mom got help with the crops from neighbors—David Hillgren, who farmed a half section (320 acres) directly north of ours and was the widower of my father's sister, Agnes; Karl Fornberg, who farmed a quarter section of 160 acres adjacent our half section to the west; and Martin Anderson, who farmed the other quarter section to the west of us. But otherwise, she could rely only on whomever of her children—three teenage girls and four boys under thirteen—were available to offer help.

My oldest sister, Georgette, who was 18 when Dad died, went off to Seattle after her high school graduation and took a job there in a munitions factory making bullets until the end of World War Two.

Eleanor, the next in line, stayed on the farm and took a year at Bethany College in Lindsborg. She then worked in nearby Salina as a telephone operator.

Ruth, the youngest of my sisters, was 15 when we lost our father. A sturdy, strong-willed, vibrant, outgoing person who enjoyed life to the fullest, she worked hard, played hard and lived hard. She stayed on the farm until she was 21, when she met Glenn Greer. A week later, they were married! Two years later, they moved to Fairbanks, Alaska.

Paul, my oldest brother, stayed home for three years after my father's death. Then, at 16, after his sophomore year of high school, he quit and hitchhiked to California with a school chum. He returned a couple of years later, but he soon married and left home for good by the time he was nineteen.

With Paul's departure for California, Johnny, at the tender age of 12, took on a more substantial role in running the farm under the guidance of Ruth and Mom. By the time he was 15 or 16, with scant help from Arnold and me, then ages twelve and nine, he was pretty much running the show as Mom's foreman.

Luckily, Johnny was a natural for farm life. In other words, he was a mechanic, a carpenter, a toolmaker, and a *fixer-upper*—the proverbial jack-of-all-trades. He quickly became the major domo. Like Mom, he was a tough, no-nonsense taskmaster. Although she did most of the cajoling and worrying about all the work that had to be done in a timely manner, it was Johnny who carried out her orders. He dragged along Arnold and me (sometimes literally kicking and screaming) to do our share.

Inevitably, Arnold and I were forced to learn many basic skills. On a farm, in addition to the motors in the trucks, tractors, balers, combines, and windmills, there are all sorts of other equipment—mowers, rakes, disks, harrows, hayracks, and binders, to name just a few. Nearly every day, something breaks down and needs fixing. Everyone becomes a mechanic out of necessity. It's a standard farmer's joke to say someone's machinery is "held together with baling wire."

We also developed three hard and fast rules. Or maybe Johnny developed them and we just obeyed them. Otherwise, there was hell to pay.

Rule Number One: Never *force* anything. If you do, something will break. Rule Number Two: Never try to do two things at the same time. If you do, you will more than likely fail at both. Rule Number Three: Never use one hand when both hands are free. If you do, the work will be slower and not as good.

Over time, I discovered that following these rules gets you through many of life's challenges.

Mom, of course, was most affected by Dad's death. Instead of living a comfortable life, she had to wage constant battle to ensure that crops were planted and harvested, that we had sufficient cows and chickens to provide milk and eggs, and that we grew enough potatoes and other vegetables. And she had to be sure to can enough of what we grew in the summer to last through the winter.

Like all mothers, she was a remarkable mix of *Jekyll and Hyde*, sweet and tart, hovering and distant, protective and stern, proud and pushy. But even with the best of intentions and amazing resolve, she could only tread water until we all grew up.

I remember the catastrophe that befell me as I was running across the Andersons' pasture to second grade class. Carrying my lunchbox and books, I tripped on a tiny stump hidden by a clump of grass. I landed hands first, and somehow my right wrist became entangled with the handle of my metal lunchbox. Snap! The bone broke like a twig.

When I arrived at school, the teacher called my mother, who took me to Doctor William Holwerda, Lindsborg's only doctor. He set my arm in a cast that had to stay on for several weeks. Once he removed it, the doctor sent the bill. His charge was five dollars. The low price embarrassed Mom, who felt we'd been given a handout. She hated being thought of as someone who'd need any kind of charity.

Against remarkable odds, she endured. That she managed to hang on to our farm and keep the family together after my father's untimely death is a wonder. That she afforded us the opportunity for humor at her expense is even more amazing.

Although Mom frequently reminded us that as a city girl how was she supposed to know all this stuff? She was always prepared to get right in the middle of things when a repair was necessary. But often we'd tease her.

"Mom," we'd say, "Would you go inside and clean the house and leave us alone?"

FARMHOUSE

The front porch of our farmhouse faced the driveway, which led to the sanded county road that marked the eastern boundary of our farm. Another two sand roads and the asphalt-paved Roxbury Road bordered the entire 640-acre section of land that included our farm and those of our neighbors, the Andersons and Fornbergs.

At the end of our driveway was a cylindrical mailbox. Wasps often built a hive in the space between its rounded surface and the board that anchored it. Opening the mailbox to retrieve the day's mail would send the wasps into action, and speed was of the essence. Needless to say, that daily task was delegated to me at a very early age. In the summertime, I dreaded it.

We had a back and front porch, both covered. We used the back porch, which faced our farmyard, as storage space for

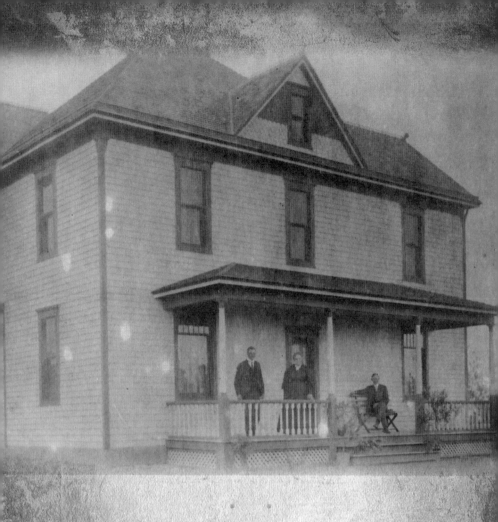

The Paulson farmhouse, rebuilt in c1915, where I was born and grew up – pictured with my father (sitting) and my Paulson grandparents our split firewood, and the dogs used it as a favorite sleeping spot, usually lying on an old, beat-up brown gunnysack. No one ever entered our house by the front door. We always went through the back porch doorway.

It opened right onto the spacious dining room, which also served as our main living room. Along with the dining table and chairs, it was furnished with a sofa (no back, just pillows resting against the wall), a large rocking chair, a sideboard and a wood-burning stove about three feet square and five feet high. At the south end of the room was a bay window, doublewide in the center. Sunlight streaming through the large window area kept the room bright and warm all year long.

The sideboard in our dining room housed Mom's best serving pieces—silverware monogrammed with an elaborately inscribed "P" and oversized white china dinner plates trimmed in silver, both used only for holiday meals. On top of the bureau were three Swedish cut-glass bowls of varying size. The drawers contained various papers and receipts deemed important or interesting.

Looking beyond the dining room from the back porch doorway, you'd see a pair of floor-to-ceiling sliding pocket doors. The doors were made of solid oak, as were the moldings that framed them and the baseboards in both rooms, and behind the doors was the parlor. It contained an upright piano, a Victrola record player, a settee and a curio cabinet. Considered our *good* room, the parlor was used only by someone playing the piano or when company *came calling*. While the dining room floor was covered with linoleum, the parlor floor was covered with a rug.

On the north wall of the dining room, opposite the bay windows, a swinging oak door led to our kitchen. The door was rarely closed, since the kitchen and dining rooms together were our primary living space. On the wall between those two rooms was a built-in cabinet.

On the dining room side, the cabinet had three large pullout drawers at the bottom and a pair of hinged glass doors at the top, all flush with the wall. On the kitchen side, a pair of solid wood doors opened onto two shelves, also accessible through the glass doors on the other side. Beneath the wood doors, there was wainscot paneling that extended around the bottom third of the other kitchen walls.

During my childhood, I heard the upper part of the cabinetry referred to exclusively as the *scopet* and until I went into high school I thought that was an English word. (It turns out that *skåpet* is Swedish for cabinet.) The *skåpet* contained our good glasses and other serving dishes, and the pullout drawers facing the dining room contained Mom's Swedish table linens. Together with the Swedish crystal and inscribed silverware, these were her most cherished possessions.

Until we got electricity in 1948, there was a coal stove in the kitchen and an icebox. There were also two tables. One was a worktable, for the preparation of food. The other, about five feet square, was where we ate all our meals except on holidays or when we had company. Both were covered in the quintessential farmers' tablecloth, red- (or blue-) and-white plaid oilcloth.

A door on the other side of the kitchen led to a small side room that was used for washing our clothes and storing all of Mom's canned foods. It was also where we kept the milk separator, which separated the milk from the cream. An upright machine, it had a very large bowl on the top. We poured the fresh strained milk into it. As we rotated the handle at high speed, the liquid passed through a set of frusto-conical disks (shaped like a cone with the top cut off). The skim milk separated from the heavier cream and each flowed into a different spout.

A second door in the kitchen led to another small room that contained a bathtub and sink, which constituted the sum and substance of bathroom space for all of us. There was no toilet. Instead, we used the outhouse. Primitive, indeed!

There was a back staircase, steep and narrow, that led into the kitchen and a less steep, wider front staircase that was covered with carpet. Tucked in under the staircases adjacent to the kitchen was a fairly large pantry. That's where Mom kept all her pots and pans, everyday dishes, glasses, and the large covered tins she used to store cookies.

A second parlor-type room was located at the foot of the front staircase and just off the door opening onto the front porch. I believe it might have been a bed/sitting room that was used by my grandparents before the house in Lindsborg was completed, but in my childhood it was used primarily as a repository for keepsakes that included old photographs, old furniture, knickknacks and sundry items from Sweden.

On the second floor were four bedrooms, including Mom's. When everyone was home, Arnold and I shared a bedroom, John and Paul shared another, and my sisters shared a third. We had a packed house!

Mom's bedroom, above the dining room, was the most spacious. It was notable for the presence of her Singer sewing machine, powered only by a foot pedal that she rocked back and forth to drive the up-and-down movement of the needle and thread. Mom's father had been a tailor, but she left Sweden at an early age, so her skill as a tailor and seamstress must just have been in her blood. She constantly and deftly altered our clothes—letting out, taking in, shortening, lengthening, attaching buttons and belt loops—and even made some of her own dresses.

Inside a large closet in Mom's bedroom, another narrow, steep staircase led to a full attic. On rainy days, Arnold and I occasionally crept up these stairs to explore the space, though what we found was not very interesting—mostly piles and piles of old, musty, dark and heavy clothing along with a smattering of old, used school workbooks and a few elementary story books. Most of the items seem to have belonged to our sisters as they grew up, and out, of their clothes and school materials.

All in all, the farmhouse accommodated our large family quite adequately, with only two drawbacks—or three, if we include the absence of plumbing. The lack of insulation meant the bedrooms in the mornings could be bitterly cold. Mom was always the first one up, stoking fires in the kitchen and dining room so that, by the time the rest of us got up at least the downstairs was warm. The presence of mice was also a constant annoyance. They seemed to live inside the walls, and setting traps was almost a daily routine.

FLORA

Farm families are interested in growing crops, either to feed their livestock or to sell to the market. We didn't pay much attention to the wildflowers unless they interfered with our productivity.

On our farm, sunflowers grew everywhere. In fact, sunflowers are the Kansas state flower—chosen, no doubt, for their ubiquity. We considered them weeds.

We never deliberately planted a single sunflower seed. In

fact, we cut them down wherever they grew. One of my earliest jobs was to chop away at the stems, using a machete-type blade as if taking a hatchet to a tree. I cut them down in our farmyard, in the pasture, in our potato patch, vegetable garden, and wheat fields.

Not only was the flower a nuisance, but also its stems and leaves were nasty to touch—slightly prickly and usually covered with a sticky, glue-like substance that oozed from pores in the stems. And, in any grove of sunflowers, there were hundreds of bees to be avoided. (In the early twenty-first century, the absence of such swarms of bees is a perplexing mystery.)

Another staple of Kansas farmland vegetation was celebrated in the song "Tumblin' Tumbleweeds." The tumbleweed has a thick profusion of tiny branches emanating from a single stem. Its branches and leaves (surrounding small flowers without petals) grow in a circular pattern in the early spring but dry out by late summer. The winds are strong enough to wrench the dried-out stems from the ground, and the rounded branches roll across open fields and roads throughout the late summer and early fall months unless they're stopped by a fence or another obstruction.

A more appealing wildflower, the morning glory, grew in the ditches adjacent to our Kansas roads. A ground-hugging vine, it produced large, white, bell-shaped flowers. As a harbinger of spring, morning glories were a welcome sight.

My grandparents had planted numerous lilac bushes in the front of our farmhouse to border the front yard. Near the center of our farmyard, but fairly close to our back porch, the ends of two steel axles from an old wagon were stuck into the ground. They formed hitching posts for horses and mules in an earlier era. In my day, when they were no longer used, a lilac bush was planted next to each.

FOUR

My first memory is of being age four, disliking it intensely, and waiting—it seemed like forever—to turn five. I don't recall any particular reason for my discontent other than the sound of the word "four" or maybe the way the word felt in my mouth. To me then (and even today) "four" had a dull and somewhat dark sound. And speaking the word required that you purse your lip downward. By contrast, I think, "five" has brightness. When you say it, your mouth is open, in a kind of smile.

When I was four, my world consisted of our farmhouse and the farmyard—a cow barn, the main barn, a machine shed, and a granary.

The cow barn had a large hayloft and was some 75 feet long. It was situated in a north-south direction and formed the southwest corner of the yard.

The main barn was located almost due south of our farmhouse. Along with the gates and pasture fencing that extended between the two barns, it marked most of the southern boundary of our farmyard. At its center peak, it was over three stories high—about 35 feet. From the highest point, the middle roof section descended halfway downward at a sharp 45-degree angle to cover over the central portion of the barn, which was about 35 feet wide. From there, the roof gently sloped outward and downward, extending about 12 feet on either side from the bottom of the center roof section.

The main barn contained several grain bins on each side

of a center drive-through that accommodated our pickup truck. A tool shop and a chicken house were on the outside of one set of grain bins. The other outer side of the main barn served as our milk shed. A series of cow stanchions were built onto almost the entire length of the interior wall of the milk shed. These stanchions were constructed as an integral unit and could accommodate eight to ten cows at once.

The cows' water tank was located near the side of the milk shed, some 60 yards south and a few yards to the west of our farmhouse. It formed a part of the northernmost boundary of the cow pasture. Although the cow tank was, at most, only about 8 feet in diameter and maybe 3 feet high and lined with a layer of "icky" green moss, it also served as my first swimming pool. It was a refreshing option on a hot summer afternoon for my eight-year-old brother, Arnold, and me.

A barbed wire fence extended west from the water tank about 30 yards, ending with a long wire gate. When swung open approximately 90 degrees, the gate could be latched to the south end of our cow barn, allowing the animals to pass into and out of the barn as they pleased. Another long wire gate was latched to a short board fence adjacent to the water tank and hinged at its opposite end to a post next to the milk shed side of our main barn. The gate and main barn continued as a boundary for the cow pasture.

To a young child, the wire gates at the water tank and cow barn provided endless joy. I swung on them, back and forth, back and forth, whenever the cows and calves were grazing down in the pasture.

It was easy to find ways to have fun on the farm, no matter what the season.

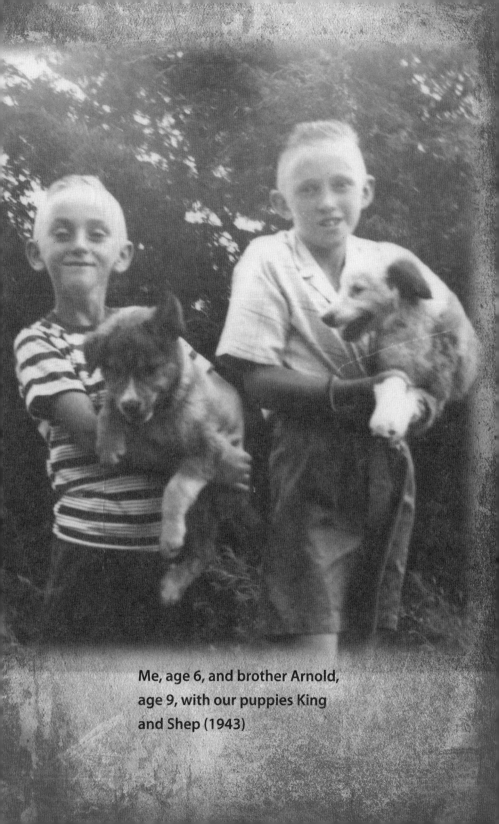

Me, age 6, and brother Arnold,
age 9, with our puppies King
and Shep (1943)

The area wasn't conducive to wintertime sledding, since most of the land around the whole Smoky Valley region consisted of gently rolling hills. But there was one good spot, Moussabacca Hill, untilled virgin pastureland about a half mile to the east of our farm. We also enjoyed trapping for rabbits, and when snow on the ground made their tracks visible, they were easy to catch and provided us with many wintertime meals.

During the cold winter months, Mom worked avidly at doing puzzles. So did we all. Much of our spare time was spent at the dining room table hovering over a pile of puzzle pieces, keeping warm thanks to a hot fire in our dining room stove. When we came inside after doing chores, Johnny, Arnold and I always took off our shoes and put our feet up against the warm sides of the stove. While sawing and splitting the logs used to stoke the fire had been agony, warming our feet and wet socks was pure ecstasy.

Between May and September, we spent untold hours under a cloudless sky doing farm work or just hanging around, dressed only in shoes, jeans, and maybe an old cap. We never wore a shirt, but that didn't give us pause. We weren't thinking about sunscreen lotion in the 40s or 50s.

I found endless ways to amuse myself. I'd climb my favorite tree, a cottonwood with no rough bark or thorns, or I'd scale the rafters of our barns and sheds. I'd locate a long thin branch on a sapling to fashion into a fishing pole, find a cork to tie to the fishing line to make into a bobber, and then hike a half-mile or so to the closest creek after digging up worms from under rocks for bait. I'd use newspaper and flour-and-water glue to put together homemade kites, with never a worry that there would be no wind in which to fly them. I'd tinker with our old bikes, patching inner tubes, tightening the handlebars, and resetting the chain. After a rainstorm, I'd climb to the top of our main barn with a piece of flat cardboard and enjoy a makeshift slipper side, careening down the wet shingles—very fast on the steep roof section, slower on the flatter, bottom section.　Or I'd play with the animals—our two dogs, King and Shep, numerous stray cats, young calves, baby pigs and young chicks.

Nature provided other diversions. After summer showers, beautiful rainbows appeared across the horizon. If only we could reach the end for that elusive *pot o' gold*! Nighttime thunderstorms produced bolts of lightning that would crackle across the sky for several seconds at a time. On the clear summer nights that were the norm, we lay on the soft grass and picked out all the constellations in the stars, most notably the Big and Little Dippers and the North Star.

"What is a star?" we wondered. "Why does it shine?" "Where did it come from?" "How does it stay in the same place in the sky each time we look up?" Youngsters throughout time have had their curiosity awakened in just such a fashion, then grown to adulthood to ponder what the famed British cosmologist Stephen Hawkings (a 45-year-survivor of ALS) calls the two Great Questions: "Why are we here?" and "How did we get here?"

But the summer I was four I was focused on less lofty thoughts. I would often be at my most favorite spot, standing on the second lowest rail of the board fencing that abutted one side of the water tank, cradling my elbows around the top rail. The sun would be bright, and a warm wind would be blowing in my face. I could see the cows and young calves coming up from the far end of the south pasture for their noontime drink of water, and all I could think of was turning five, finally able to rid myself forever of that dreaded label—"four"!

ONE-ROOM SCHOOLHOUSE

At last, I turned five, but I was doomed to further disappointment. Without warning, one morning Johnny and Arnold trotted off to school and Mom wouldn't let me go with them because I was too young. When I learned I would have to wait a year, I cried my eyes out. Nothing Mom said could console me. (I had an entire year of complete carefree freedom ahead of me, and I was distraught. Sometimes we just don't recognize a good thing when it's in front of us.)

Our Smoky Hill Township School was a one-room schoolhouse about a mile west of our farmhouse, across a couple of fields and a pasture. We walked to school unless the temperature dipped below zero. My brothers and sisters all went there for the first eight grades, and I went for the first five.

The schoolhouse was located on approximately an acre of land. At one end were two outdoor toilets spaced apart on opposite sides of the schoolyard. At the other were a set of swings and a teeter-totter, both of which I thoroughly enjoyed. In between these landmarks was open grass-covered space, perfect for softball or touch football. There was also a small coal shed on the grounds.

At the entrance to the schoolhouse building was a small hall, about 10 x 10, where we hung our coats and left our lunch boxes in locker-type cubbies.

The main room was about 70 feet long and 30 feet wide. Near the doorway stood the coal stove that provided heat in winter, and in front of it were four rows of desks graduated in size to fit everyone from a first- to an eighth-grader. Directly in front of three of the desk rows was a long bench.

At the rear of the room were the cabinets that held our library, and beneath them were two large, built-in tables for art projects. Windows lined the two side walls.

At the front end of the room was a small stage, raised up about one foot. The teacher sat at a desk in the middle of it, and a blackboard extended across the wall behind her.

On the floor next to one side of the stage was an upright piano, its back up against the side wall of the building, Directly opposite the piano, a doorway led to a kitchen about 20 feet square. We could wash our hands and get a drink of water in the kitchen, but it was used primarily for community social events.

The kitchen extended outward perpendicular to the main schoolhouse. Its peaked roof was considerably lower than the roof of the main building. We'd play a game of catch over that roof, yelling "*Alley oop*" as the ball was heaved. The receiver couldn't see the ball until it cleared the rooftop, and the challenge was to catch it before it hit the ground.

When I entered first grade at the Smokey Hill School, Arnold was in fourth and Johnny was in eighth. Altogether, there were 14 students, including the Hanson children: Lloyd Ray and Lola, who lived directly south of our farm; the Finneys: Raymond, Anita and Rosalie, who lived two miles south and slightly west of us; the Patricks: Arlen, Richard and Barbara, who lived two miles to the north, just on the other side of David Hillgren's farm; the Nordbergs: Lloyd and Mildred; and Verlyn Gabrielson.

Though it must have been a challenge for the teacher

to teach all eight grade levels in one room, learning in that environment had some marvelous advantages. In the course of the day, each class was brought forward to sit on the long front bench just in front of the teacher's desk. Particularly when math or history was the subject, I was able to follow work being taught at two or three grade levels above mine. By the time it was appropriate for me to tackle a subject, I had a good idea of what was coming and could easily grasp what was taught.

GATHERINGS

Mom was the treasurer of the school board and held meetings at the schoolhouse. It also served as a social gathering place for parents as well as nearby farmers and relatives. On such occasions, it was a beehive of activity, with ladies setting up their dishes of food, unwrapping cakes, pies and cookies, and percolating gallons of coffee.

My mother was usually in charge of making the coffee for the adults at school functions. She brewed it in two-gallon coffee pots, and her flavoring trick was to crack an egg right on top of the coffee grounds with each new full pot.

A Halloween party was the first exciting social event of each school year. The adults turned the kerosene lamps low and hung heavy curtains to create a dark walk-through maze crisscrossed with spider webbing, luminous skeletons, bats and insects and other creatures of the night. Older kids stationed behind the curtains added to the scariness of the maze journey by producing blood-curdling screams.

A batch of fresh, homemade cakes would be spread out on a table for the winners of the cakewalk. The cakewalk is

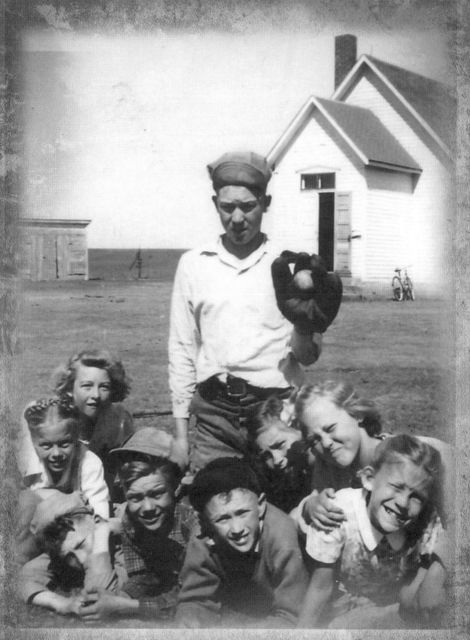

Smoky Hill Schoolhouse (background), with classmates Arlen Patrick (top, with ball and glove), Lola Hanson, Mildred Nordberg, Barbara Patrick (middle row), me (hidden on far left), Anita Finney, Dickie Patrick, Raymond Finney, my brother, Arnold, and Roslaie Finney (bottom row)

like musical chairs. While a pianist played, participants walked single file in a big circle past a blindfolded kid who held a broom by the straw end (with the pole handle up in the air.) When the music stopped, everyone froze, and the child with the broom would drop the handle. Whoever it touched was a winner.

The evening's festivities also included bobbing for apples in a washtub filled with water. And frequently, the Crazy Ridge Cowboys, a local country music group, would perform.

Mom was also an active member of two ladies' clubs, the Laugh-a-Lot Club and the Mount Hope Community Club. Each met once a month at the farmhouse of one of the members, and I recall get-togethers during the summer months. Between the ages of four to nine, I accompanied Mom on several occasions.

These club day afternoons were great fun. There were always two or three other kids my age, and we'd go off to explore machine sheds and visit the animals—sometimes baby calves, new kittens or puppies. And there were always deviled eggs, lots of good sandwiches, and peanut butter cookies.

Martin and Edith Anderson's farm was the one I most enjoyed visiting because Martin was an inveterate junk collector. Every spare inch of his barns, every nook and every cranny was filled with machine paraphernalia of indescribable breadth. Old and mostly rusty, the collection included axles, iron wheels, rods, bolts, springs, metal seats off old tractors— anything and everything.

Still more old and rusty miscellaneous metal machine parts were stacked outside in neat piles all over the place between the outer sheds and barns. The farmyard was virtually a maze of pathways between piles of this stuff. I have no idea how or from where Martin could have acquired so much useless junk. But for visiting kids, it made for great games of hide-and-seek!

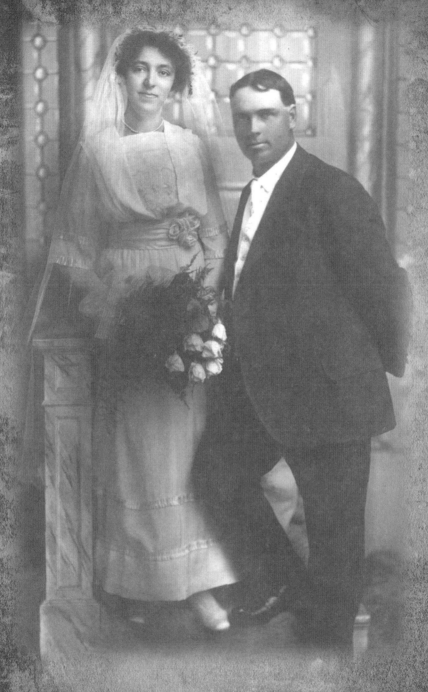

My aunt Agnes Paulson Hillgren and
husband David Hillgren, married c1920

DAVID

My mother enjoyed the frequent company of our neighbor David Hillgren.

He was a widower. His wife—my father's sister Agnes—had died in 1934, five years before my dad, of causes that no one, including Mom, seemed able to explain.

David's farm was just to the north of ours across Roxbury Road. David had posted a sign at the entrance to his driveway that read "Sunnyhill Farm." That was an apt description of the picturesque farmhouse and farm buildings, atop a large knoll facing south and surrounded by a ring of evergreens.

His driveway was a good quarter mile long. It dipped down from the Roxbury Road before rising to reach the house and outer buildings, and continued in a great circle around the farmhouse, connecting his machine sheds, garages and barns.

David was a fastidious *neatnik*. All his farm machinery was carefully stowed away in the machine sheds, and in between the sheds and other buildings was closely cropped buffalo grass. His Model A Ford coupe, circa 1925, was immaculate. He drove it throughout my high school years and for several years thereafter. Although he often wore bib overalls, they seemed to be pressed, and his high-topped boots were always shined.

David was a bit portly and walked with the aid of a cane and somewhat bent over. One of his horses had given a bad kick to the knee that never healed.

Throughout my school years in Lindsborg, David would drive up to our place on a late afternoon and park right by our back porch, his customary stogie in his mouth. He rarely came inside. Instead, Mom climbed into his Model A and there they sat and talked, quietly and amiably, for hours.

WATER

We had four water wells on our farm, with two separate windmills. The windmills were the classic design frequently depicted in a farming landscape: a four-legged, braced iron framework tapering upwards 20 or 25 feet from a six-foot square at the bottom to a three-foot-square at the top. On the top platform, the fan blades were mounted on an axle that turned a gearbox, converting the rotary motion to reciprocal motion in order to pump water out of the well.

One windmill was located in our cow pasture. Pipes led to one tank right beside it and to another in our yard near the barns. A second windmill in the center of our yard also brought water to two wells. One, located next to the house, supplied drinking and cooking water. The other well, meant to collect rainwater for bathing, was located under our house next to the kitchen.

All our house water had to be hand pumped into a bucket and carried inside. We all hated this chore, which was of course never-ending. We needed water to drink, to wash dishes, to wash clothes, to boil potatoes, to take a bath, to wash our hands and faces, and so on. The job of pumping yet another bucket went usually to the low man on the totem pole. That would be me. "Gul dang it, not again, not already?" I'd think. "Gee whiz!"

I never gave a second thought to the composition of our water. No one ever came to test it. We just drank what came out of the spout. Moreover, our drinking water pump used small iron cups attached to an iron cog chain that pulled up the water from the well. Obviously, everything was rusted from sitting in the water. I drank the same water as our cows. We all did. Somehow, we survived. The iron was probably good for us.

When I eventually arrived in the District of Columbia and later in New York, all the dentists I visited commented on the hardness of my teeth and wanted to know where I had grown up. Whatever else our Kansas well water contained, it was apparently loaded with beneficial minerals.

TEAMWORK

On our farm, everyone had to pitch in. We grumbled and moaned, like all kids, but the chores always got done somehow.

I was only six or seven when I was given my first farm responsibility—gathering the eggs and feeding and watering the chickens. When I got older, I joined Johnny and Arnold in milking the cows. Arnold and I usually ran the milk separator in tandem, one of us pulling and the other pushing on the crank to bring it up to speed to begin operating. Meanwhile, Johnny would be feeding the baby calves that had been weaned from their mothers. Then we all worked at mixing the skim milk with bran and corn meal and feeding it to the pigs, the best of which would be entered in the next 4-H County fair.

If we were late milking the cows, likely on a Saturday morning after a Friday night football game, Mom might get exasperated. "It's a good thing I never learned how to milk a cow or I guess I'd be doing that too!" she'd say. Instead, she took on the responsibility for doing the wash along with the cooking, the cleaning, and the myriad other household chores.

Washdays in the farmhouse were very exciting to me when I was young. There was a great bustle of activity as Mom gathered up all the dirty clothes, separated them into several piles around the kitchen floor, heated up water in kettles on top of the stove, and then started up the small (but loud) motor under the washing machine. Amid the commotion and noise, I huddled under the kitchen table, taking in everything from a safe distance.

A clothes wringer was mounted on top of the washing machine. As I got older, my job was to catch each piece of clothing as Mom cranked it through the rolls of the wringer and then to place in a basket. When all the wash was finished, I helped her carry the baskets out to the clotheslines. Once I was tall enough, I pulled a rag along each line to clean off any dust or dirt before the clothes were pinned up to dry. Thanks to the sun and the ever-present wind, the clothes dried in no time at all. Even after we had electricity, we never had a clothes dryer on the farm. Just as well, I think. Nothing else has the sweet smell of a piece of clothing washed and then dried in the sun.

In the winter, washdays were not so pleasant. We'd have to stand in the bitter wind to pump buckets of water, and then we'd lug them into the house, getting splashed along the way. Mom would hang the wrung-out clothes on an inside clothesline rigged up to stretch across the kitchen. Heat for drying came from our trusty kitchen coal stove, and, in the days before we were wired for electricity, the coal stove also heated the irons.

Having spent a day washing and drying the sheets, pants, and dress shirts, Mom then would spend several evenings ironing them. Back then, wash-and-wear clothing didn't exist, and Johnny, Arnold and I together produced a lot of shirts.

It was something of a performance. With a bit of a show that was quite out of character for her, Mom would pluck an iron off the stovetop to test if it were ready. She'd dip her fingertips in a cup of water, then snap her fingers close to the bottom of the iron, and by the sound of the water vaporizing, gauge if it were hot enough. She'd turn out perfectly starched collars and cuffs and perfectly flattened material in between. Even the cloth around the buttons was carefully circled and smoothed out.

When we went off to college, we still brought home our dirty shirts on school breaks for Mom to deal with. Maybe we were just boys being boys, but none of us ever offered to iron anything. Milking and feeding the animals were our jobs, and the washing, cooking and ironing were hers. Not a bad deal for either of us, I'd say. We didn't give much thought to how the jobs were parceled out. We just understood that working together was necessary.

We did our share as best as we could, and the older we children got, the more we did. Everyone speaks of the value of learning teamwork from playing sports like basketball or football. I played those sports. But I think my real grounding in learning the value of teamwork and cooperation came from our farm work.

WAR RATIONS

I remember very little about World War II. I have a vague recollection of seeing a newspaper headline about the war ending in 1945, but I was just eight years old.

The only truly vivid memory I have of that time is learning about the death of my cousin Carl Helge Jacobson, though I have no memory of Carl himself. The youngest son of my father's sister, Helga, Carl Helge was serving in the Navy as a gunner on the cruiser ship U.S.S. Savannah, then on maneuvers in the Mediterranean, firing against German shore defenses in

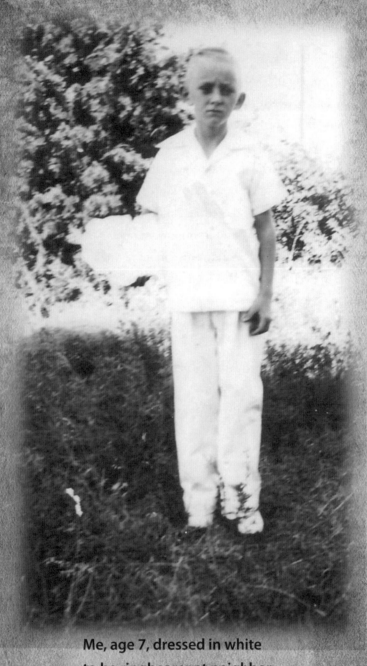

Me, age 7, dressed in white
to be ringbearer at neighbor
Jane Anderson's wedding

Salemo Bay, Sicily. He was killed instantly on September 11, 1943, when a German bomb landed directly on the gun turret he was manning. A total of 197 men died in the attack. Needless to say, we paid a very sad visit to my grandfather's house in Lindsborg when Aunt Helga got the news.

I also recall a lot of airplane activity in the sky above our farm. We were under a flight path for the Smoky Hill Air Force base, a busy place during the war years. Occasionally, a jet fighter plane would zoom low over our fields and tip its wings. Johnny would say, "Guess that's one of the Koons boys, waving to their parents." The Koons' sons were both pilots, and their farm was a few miles southeast of us.

I remember hearing about the Japanese *kamikaze* pilots flying their Zero fighter planes (manufactured by Mitsubishi) into our Navy ships, deliberately blowing themselves up for the glory of the Japanese Emperor. And I recall the German phrase "Achtung," probably from comic books.

As for the war's effect on our daily life, I remember that we could buy only oleomargarine as a substitute for butter. It was white and tasted like lard, and it came with a packet of yellow food coloring. Although the yellow color made the *oleo* look better, it still tasted like lard. No wonder that our freshly churned butter was especially delicious by comparison.

I remember gas rationing as another issue, but it had no impact on us because farmers were exempted. We bought gas in 50-gallon drums, usually two at a time, so could always dump four or five gallons into our car for the 12-mile trip to McPherson, the county seat, or Salina, a larger town about 20 miles away.

Gasoline at the pump in those days was 25 or 30 cents a

gallon. For years, even up to the time when I began to drive, my mother would pull up to the pump and say, "A dollar's worth, please!" If occasionally she felt flush with money, she asked for two dollars' worth of gas. We never filled up!

PLAYMATES

We had many enjoyable times visiting the children of our neighboring farm families.

The Andersons were best friends to our family. Their older children, Jack and Jane, were contemporaries of my sisters and my oldest brother Paul. Jack Anderson eventually took a job with the federal agency that would bring electricity to the farmlands in 1948, and I served as ring bearer at Jane's wedding.

Their youngest child was some ten years older than I. Leviva was an invalid, confined to a wheelchair for her whole life. She suffered from a birth defect that left her legs useless, and I remember how weak she seemed to me when I was an 8-year-old. Still, Leviva was able to use her hands and could speak.

Sometimes during my years in the one-room schoolhouse, I would walk to the Andersons' house after school, along with the Finney girls, Anita and Rosalie, and do cross-stitch sewing with Leviva. I guess we were good company for Leviva, but our hand towels, tablecloths and pillowcases were quite amateurish. Because Mom's father had been a tailor in Sweden and she was a gifted seamstress, perhaps she thought I would have some innate ability with a needle and thread. No such luck.

Arnold and I also spent a lot of time with the Finneys, because the girls were close to my age and their brother Raymond was Arnold's age (and remained his good friend through their college years). It was an easy bike ride to their farm, which had a small creek nearby for fishing and a huge cottonwood tree that was perfect for climbing. Best of all, Mrs. Finney always seemed to have freshly baked cookies and lemonade to offer Arnold and me before we pedaled home.

One year, just before school opened at Smoky Hill, we went on an outing with the Patricks of which I have a particularly vivid memory. They invited Mom, Arnold and me to ride with them to the State Fair in Hutchinson, located about 40 miles away. On the way, we witnessed a true Kodak moment. On the outskirts of Hutch, we were driving past a number of small houses clumped together, kind of a shantytown, when the door of one burst open and a man ran out at full speed. Directly behind, traveling just as fast, came a woman waving a frying pan over her head. We missed the ending, but that scene came straight out of a cartoon strip. Priceless!

COWS AND CALVES

Having a herd of cows is a mixed blessing for a farmer. The milk is great—it provides a growing family with all the milk the kids can drink plus extra to sell and also cream that can be used, sold, or made into butter. But the obligation to milk the cows day and night, with never a break, can be a heavy stone to carry, no matter how few cows are in the herd.

Our mornings were a frenzy of activity. Get up, put on old clothes, go to the barn to put out a small cup of corn meal in the stanchion for each cow, call the cows in from pasture, milk them, and carry five or six gallons back to the house. Put aside some for drinking, run the rest through the separator to divide off the cream, then carry the skim milk out to the pig pen, mix it with bran, corn meal and other grains to make a slurry, and "slop the hogs" by pouring the heavy mixture into their trough. Feed extra milk to three or more calves, then wash up, dress for school, have a bowl of cereal (with fresh cream, never milk, thank you), and walk—mostly run—a mile across two fields and a pasture to the schoolhouse. Whew! How did we ever have time for school? And come evening, the process would have to be repeated—every day of every week of every month of every year.

I began to help with the milking of our seven or eight cows starting when I was nine or ten. Learning to hand milk a cow is an art in and of itself. You must wear something like a baseball cap on your head and be carrying a clean pail in one hand and a small stool in the other.

Then you have to make three nearly simultaneous moves: Crouch down and place your head firmly into the cow's flank (the soft spot just in front of the upper portion of the hind leg), put the stool under you with one hand, and settle onto the stool while using the other hand to put the pail between your legs. As you begin to milk, you have to press your left forearm against the cow's hind leg and squeeze your legs tightly together to firmly hold the pail between them.

These precautions are necessary because when the cow's udder and teats are full of milk, the first touch and squeeze of the teats can be slightly painful for the cow. Pressing your head into its flank and your arm against its leg tells the cow to resist the urge to kick. But occasionally the cow still lets go with a good kick, sending the pail flying. Not only do you lose whatever milk your efforts might already have produced, but also you have to start all over again with a clean pail.

Occasionally, I'd have to help wean a three-month-old calf— teach it to drink milk from a bucket. This, too, is no easy task. You hold the calf tightly against the side of the pen with one knee, put your hand in the bucket of milk, and get the calf to suck the milk from your fingers. With your fingers still in the calf's mouth, you shove its nose into the bucket and let it drink while still sucking on your fingers. After a few moments, you pull out your fingers while pushing down on the calf's head. It will buck a few times with its hind legs. A front leg may end up in the bucket, a bucket or two may spill, and milk will be splashed all over your clothes, but after two or three sessions, you'll have succeeded in teaching the calf to drink from a bucket.

TOWN POOL

Some of my most enjoyable summer outings were the Sunday afternoons we spent at the McPherson town swimming pool. We didn't go on a regular basis, which made the few visits there that much more memorable. I certainly will never forget the occasion when, at age nine or ten, I nearly lost my life.

The design of the McPherson Pool was unique and interesting. It was a series of concentric circles. The outer ring was a concrete walkway surrounded by grass and benches. The next ring was about 8 feet wide and filled with sand, a delight for the youngest kids. Inside the sand ring was the first ring of shallow water, separated from the sand by just a small, rounded hump. The shallow water gently sloped from a few inches to about 3-1/2 feet deep, where there was a sturdy iron fence consisting of vertical rods about 4 inches apart. Inside the iron fence, the bottom of the pool sloped again, this time sharply, to a depth of about 12 to 15 feet. About every 15 feet or so, an opening in the fence allowed access from the shallow to the deep-water area.

In the center of the deep water, a circular platform provided the base for several diving boards that jutted out over the water. They ranged in height from a low of three feet to a high of ten feet. The deep-water ring was about 20 to 25 feet across, wide enough to ensure that no diver could mistakenly be thrown against the fencing.

Naturally, the fence openings to the deep water were tempting to me, even though I could manage only a lame version of the dog paddle. On that near-fateful day, I foolishly went through one opening, pulling myself along in the deep water while clinging to the inside of the fence. Though I occasionally let go of the fence to paddle, I kept close by. Then, in an instant, it was out of reach, and I was floundering, out of my depth.

As I began to sink, I caught a breath and continued to paw at the water. When I saw the bottom of the fencing rods, I made one last desperate lunge. Somehow, I got my fingertips around one and pulled myself up out of the water. I quickly got out of the pool, ran to a bench and vowed "Never again!"

Three years later, Lindsborg built its own municipal pool in a conventional rectangular design. I learned to swim well enough to pass a lifesaving course, and I worked as a pool lifeguard for three summers during my college years. To this day, I can't recall seeing another swimming pool designed like the McPherson Pool.

Although aesthetically attractive, it was fraught with hazards. Unsuspecting or rash non-swimmers like me could easily pass through the fence openings to the deep water. The circular arrangement made it hard for lifeguards to monitor the swimmers from the center platform. Finally, springboard diving boards are exceedingly dangerous, since a novice diver can be thrown great distances by the spring action of the board. Considering the crazy stunts young adults are prone to try without considering possible consequences, it was amazing that the McPherson Pool sustained no unhappy incidents. Though it was conventionally designed, the Lindsborg pool, as it turned out, would be less fortunate.

PIGS

A special word for pigs, my buddies! We always raised a bevy of pigs. They were registered Duroc Reds that were easily trained to respond when they were scratched behind the ears or their snouts were rubbed. So long as their bellies were full, they were very content and would grunt softly, making a sound not unlike a cat's purring.

Our sows would deliver an average of six to eight piglets in a litter. When a sow was close to giving birth, we placed her in her own small pen where we had attached a railing around the bottom, eight to ten inches from the floor. The tiny piglets could run under the railing and not be accidentally crushed by the hulk of the sow as she lay down—more accurately, made a quick flop—and stretched out fully to allow the entire litter could feed at one time from both rows of her teats.

When I was younger than ten, I could ride on the backs of my pigs once they were about a year old.

We always had one or two pigs to enter in the annual 4-H County Fair where they had to be *shown*—led around in a

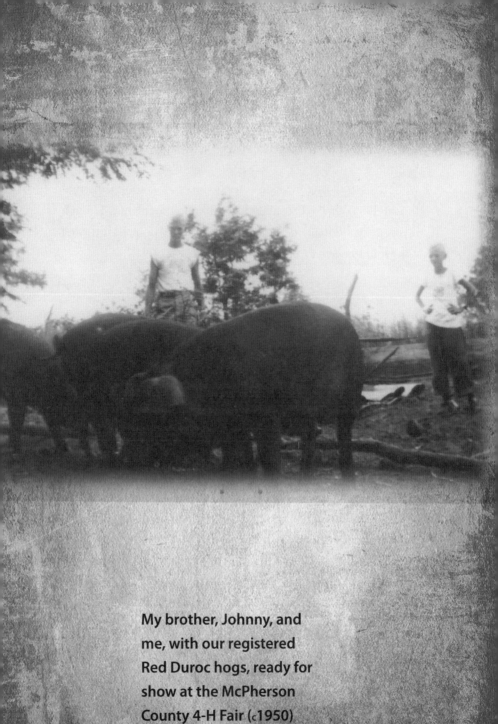

My brother, Johnny, and me, with our registered Red Duroc hogs, ready for show at the McPherson County 4-H Fair (c1950)

ring, then stopped before a judge with both front and back legs aligned, much like competitors in a dog show. But with pigs, there was no halter or leash. For some kids, the event involved more chasing the animals around than stopping and showing.

Johnny was the best in our family at showing our pigs. Since the pig had to be washed and brushed constantly during showing, Johnny always had a brush in one hand. Whenever his pig sought to move when he should be still, Johnny used the back of the brush to rap it on the nose. He trained his pigs very well.

Contrary to their reputation for slovenliness, pigs use a special corner of their pen exclusively for their toileting. No doubt that perception arose because they constantly root in the dirt with their snouts and like elephants they love to wallow in mud holes to cool off. But they're just muddy, not dirty.

One early winter, Johnny built a lean-to about 40 inches high and 12 feet long in the pigpen, and he then draped gunnysacks across the open side of the lean-to facing south. Inside the lean-to, I spread out a couple bales of fresh straw. One particularly cold, snowy and windy day, the pigs were all lounging close together with mounds of straw half-covering them and also in between. While the snow and wind whistled outside, it was so warm and cozy in the lean-to that I just picked out a spot between two pigs, curled up and took a little snooze!

FOOD

Food was a big deal to us boys.

Nothing in my farm life was more welcome than Mom's announcement that she would bake bread. There's nothing better than fresh, piping hot bread just out of the oven and

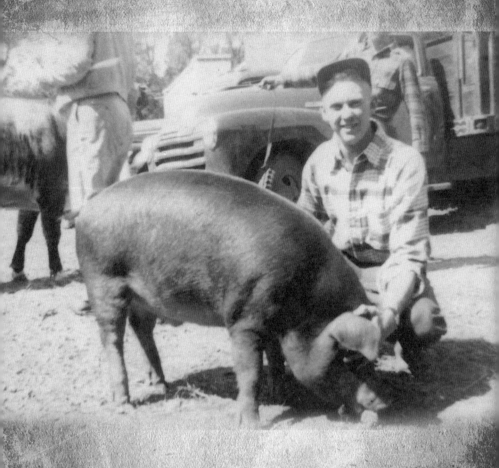

My brother, Johnny, at
Kansas State Free Fair,
showing his Blue Ribbon
Red Duroc, Reserve
Champion pig (1949)

homemade butter. But like every farm chore, making it was not an easy task. Mom had to mix the dough, put it in a milk bucket and wait for it to rise, knead it, return it to the bucket and wait for a second rise, then knead it again. Only then could it go into the oven.

While Mom was working on the bread, I would churn up a batch of fresh butter. Our churn was a jug about two and a half feet high and a foot in diameter. The paddle, mounted on the end of a long pole, was a circular disc full of holes. We'd pour a gallon or so of cream into the churn, slip the paddle pole through the hole in the lid, and then place the lid on the churn. My job was to run the paddle up and down long enough—about 35 to 40 minutes—to turn that gallon of cream into two pounds of butter.

The staple items on our table were chicken, pork and potatoes, supplemented, especially in the summer, by a great assortment of vegetables. These would include tomatoes, beans, peas, squash, asparagus, onions, beets, and carrots, plus lettuce, cabbage, and cauliflower, which we grew in abundance. In season, we'd also have watermelon and cantaloupe, strawberries, mulberries, peaches, grapes, and plums. Though we didn't grow apples, pears, or oranges, we bought them by the bushel. To carry the vegetables and fruits into the winter, my mother spent several intense days canning as much as possible.

We found that the quickest way to plant potatoes was to plow a furrow, place potato buds near the bottom at 18-inch intervals, then plow over that furrow and repeat the planting in the next one. We usually planted at least 1-1/2 acres of potatoes each spring season. You had to cultivate the plants by hand, a job that fell mostly to Arnold and me, each carrying a hoe. It was backbreaking work.

When the potato plants were nearing maturity, there were always goodly crops of potato bugs to reckon with. Actually, we considered the challenge fun. We'd fill old coffee cans with a cup or two of gasoline, hand-pick the bugs off the plants, drop them in the gasoline and then set the gas on fire, watching the bugs fry with a sizzle and crack. Though perhaps a little ghoulish, it was effective.

As much as I considered each of our pigs a pet, every fall our local butcher slaughtered one of them— right in our farmyard. The butcher was led to the pigpen. When the designated pig was pointed out to him, he shot it between the eyes, and then he slit its throat open. Its blood would be drained into a kitchen pan. My mother later would add flour to the blood and bake it in the oven. She'd cut baked "blood pudding" into squares and serve it, usually with scrambled eggs, at breakfast. We didn't give it a second thought, but I don't think I could eat that dish today!

After the pig had been bled, it was dragged to the center of our yard. The butcher set up a large wooden tripod and then hoisted the carcass up by the hind legs so the pig hung upside down. Any remaining blood in the pig oozed out of the animal's slit throat.

The butcher then quickly set about carving the hide off the body of the pig. When it was fully skinned, he wrapped the whole carcass in a clean cloth and loaded it into his pickup truck to take to his shop in Lindsborg. There the carcass was cut into roasts, pork chops, bacon strips and so on. Ultimately it was stored in a large freezer room that held dozens of three-foot-square, wire-enclosed bins, each holding a store of meat for families in the community. A trip to the meat locker was always quick. With the temperature at about 20° Fahrenheit in the locker, it was no place to lollygag!

In the farmyard, the chickens ruled, simply because there were so many of them. Remembering the location of all their nests in my daily round of egg collecting was a challenge.

My mother always ordered 100 new chicks every year, usually in the early spring. The chicks were shipped by railroad, and they came in boxes about three feet square and perhaps eight inches high. They were partitioned into quarter sections, with 25 chicks in each. Small holes punched in the cardboard box allowed air inside. Each quarter section contained two small cups wedged into the outer wall, one for food and one for water.

We raised our chicks in a separate building behind the main barn. The chicken house contained two brooders for keeping the chicks warm. Each brooder contained a heating element and a large circular hood extending close to the floor.

One chilly night, when I was about eight, tragedy struck our brood of young chicks. The door to the dining room had been closed to keep the kitchen warm, and we had made popcorn on the hot top of the kitchen stove. Ruth, Mom, John, Arnold and I were playing cards at the kitchen table. The game was friendly but spirited, and all of us were deeply absorbed in it. When it was over, everyone got up from the table and stretched, ready for bed. Then, I threw open the door to the dining room. Through the window was a shocking sight. The chicken house was completely ablaze!

The pleasant, fun-filled mood of the evening turned to one of sadness and despair. The fire was so far gone that there was just nothing to do but watch the chicken house burn to the

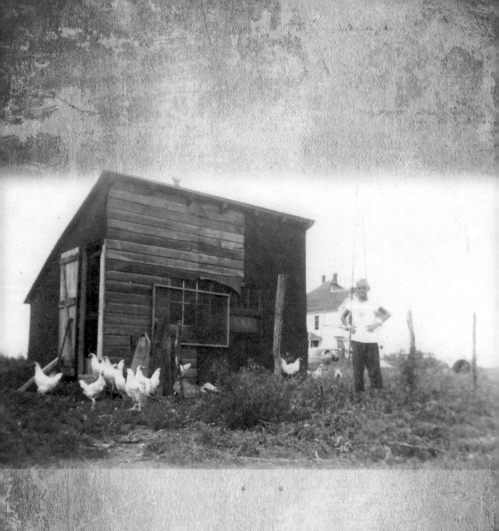

Me with my chickens and
the chickenhouse that
burned down (c1948)

ground. Somehow, one of the brooders had malfunctioned.

After that terrible accident, we never rebuilt the chicken house. Another era ended in the Paulson family history.

4-H

The 4-H credo is to pledge oneself to better thinking, better living, better helping for others, and better use of one's abilities, and the H's refer to Head, Heart, Hands and Health. Though today its purpose has expanded to include youth everywhere, the organization was originally created for farm youth.

Johnny was a star in the McPherson County 4-H. Over the years, he won many awards, including Best Public Speaker for an address he had worked up on the qualities of leadership. He was awarded the title of McPherson County Wheat King for collecting the most bushels of wheat from area farmers for donation to the World Hunger Organization. (Some farmers actually refused to give even a single bushel!). One year, he bought a new suit and tie and won the countywide title in the 4-H clubs as "Best-Dressed Young Man." (Mom, Arnold and I had a good laugh at that one!)

Naturally, Johnny's successes inspired his brothers to become involved in 4-H activities, which included entering various competitions at the annual county fair. One of them challenged you to give a three-to-five minute "how to" demonstration about any aspect of farm life. The point of the exercise was to give young people experience at public speaking, and the theory was that focusing on a specific topic and using props would help calm their inevitable jitters.

One year, our club leader suggested that Arnold and I

work together to demonstrate the proper way to file a hoe. Could anything be simpler? The two of us worked out our respective roles and collected our props. I believe I held the hoe while Arnold wielded the file. We showed the audience that you place the file at an angle to the back edge of the hoe and file in one direction only. Filing back and forth, we explained, would dull the surface you have just sharpened. And that was it.

With some chagrin, I realize today that the Paulson boys failed to recognize the commercial value of simple demonstrations. Look at how Martha Stewart has become a multi-millionaire by showing millions of women how to perform such simple tasks as trimming a window shade, tying a decorative bow, decorating for Christmas, setting a table, and putting together a picnic lunch.

We had the savvy. We knew how to sharpen a hoe. But we didn't know how to *monetize* our skills, as they say today. I guess we were just born too soon! Perhaps we also needed to find a more compelling subject than how to file a hoe.

WIRED UP

The Rural Electrification Act of 1948 was a wondrous milestone, a major change in our way of life. I was 11 years old. The first indication that something was happening was that Mom began picking out lighting fixtures. Shortly after that, several fellows came to the house and wired us for electricity. They even put up a telephone pole near our windmill and ran a line to it so we could have a yard light as well as a shared telephone line.

Since I had begun to spend more time studying, the arrival of electricity was especially well-timed for me. I no longer had to squint and strain my eyes in the dim, flickering light of the kerosene lamp. Kerosene lamps were also dangerous. Shortly before we got electricity, I had been carrying a kerosene lamp down the stairs when I tripped and fell to the bottom. Although the glass chimney flew off and shattered, I somehow held onto the burning lamp. My leg was bruised, as was my ego, but I had narrowly averted a potentially disastrous fire.

With the coming of electricity, we also replaced our kitchen coal stove with an electric range; though Mom later said the electric oven just didn't measure up to the one in the coal stove. We abandoned the biweekly chore of bringing home a 100-pound ice block and hoisting it up into the upper chamber of the icebox. We no longer had to chip slivers of ice from the block. Now we had a refrigerator and ice cubes!

And we got a radio. Our family often gathered around it on early Sunday evenings to listen to the exploits of Sergeant Preston of the Canadian Mounted Police and his ever-faithful dog King, The Green Hornet, and The Shadow. For years I was enraptured by the story lines, the strong voices of the lead characters, and the fascinating sound effects. What listener can forget the eerie squeak of the closing door, the devilish laugh, and the sonorous voice asking, "Who knows what evil lurks behind the door? ...The Shadow knows!"

But even after we got electricity, we hadn't thoroughly modernized. We never did get a television set. And we retained the four-party telephone line throughout all my high school years. The number of rings indicated which party was receiving the call. The shared telephone system was the source of much amusement, speculation, consternation and mischief.

"I wonder who's calling the Fornbergs at this time of

night?"

"Gee, how can anyone talk so long?"

"Why hasn't Eleanor called? Is the line still busy?"

Of course, I did my share of tying up the line. When a classmate (usually Martha or Loren) and I were studying by phone, we were often interrupted by someone on my party line or theirs, "Please get off the line. I have to make a call!"

The telephone we used, a wooden box mounted to our kitchen wall, was a classic of the period. On one side of the box was a U-shaped clip that held a heavy earphone; on the other was a little handle that could be cranked. To make a call, you lifted the earphone off the clip, pressed it against your ear, and turned the handle two or three rotations. That *rang up* an operator sitting at a large switchboard in Salina.

"Number, please?" she'd ask.

You spoke the number directly into the horn piece, a foghorn-shaped piece of metal that stuck out from the center of the box, and the operator manually connected you on her switchboard with the desired number.

Except for the two-way radio on the wrist of the comic book detective Dick Tracy, this crude telephone system was the most modern we could imagine. None of us dreamed of a wireless cell phone, computer design was in its very infancy, and television was still not available to most of America. The contrast between the telephone of my childhood and the cell phones of today is symbolic of the striking technological advances made in the past 60 years.

IMPASSES

Weather conditions often made it difficult to get our cars on the road.

Our farmhouse and yard were at the top of a gentle rolling hill, so the driveway, about an eighth of a mile long, was on a slight incline. It ran into a county road that was sanded and maintained by the McPherson County Roads Department. Half a mile north, the sand road intersected with the Roxbury Road, running east-west. Two miles west on Roxbury was US Highway 81, a two-lane concrete road. Driving north on 81 for half a mile, you'd arrive in Lindsborg.

We never sanded our driveway until years after Johnny came back from Korea. All through my school years, two tire ruts in our driveway zigzagged all the way from top to bottom. When it rained, getting up the driveway was a challenge. The ruts were five or six inches deep, but however much a driver tried to straddle them, his wheels almost inevitably would slip back into the ruts, and the car would be stuck in time. The driveway inclined enough so that the tires would only spin in place. Someone would get out and push. If that didn't help, the driver would back up in the ruts all the way to the bottom and try once again. Sometimes we just left the car at the bottom of the driveway and walked up to the house.

Winter cold presented other problems. Every car we owned was second or third hand. In really cold weather, below about 10° Fahrenheit, the car would never start. To get it going, we would first start up the tractor by manually cranking the crankshaft, then hook up a chain to the bumper of the car, and use the tractor to tow the car. The trick was to pick up a little speed, and then "drop" the clutch with the gear engaged to turn

The Paulson farmhouse
and driveway (June 1967)

over the crankshaft. Usually the car would start after one or two attempts, but a lot of consternation surrounded the whole process.

Wind created issues year round. In late summer, winds would blow tumbleweeds across open fields and roads, and in winter they would blow and drift snow into great tufts that were impassable with a car or truck. Whenever there was a snowstorm of any significant force, our driveway was always drifted over. There wasn't much weather forecasting in those days. Being snowed in always caught us by surprise. Usually, we just waited a few days until the county snowplow dug us out. Sometimes, we could drive over frozen fields blown clear by the wind to get egress onto the Roxbury Road and from there, to get to Lindsborg.

LINDSBORG

Lindsborg proper is primarily located just north of the Smoky Hill River. US Highway 81 forms its eastern border, running north and south as it passes the town.

Approximately three blocks to the west of 81 are the Union Pacific railroad tracks, which arrive in Lindsborg from the south and west. Until I was in high school, passenger trains stopped in Lindsborg, permitting train passage direct to Denver or Chicago, and all points in between.

The Farmers' Union, where local farmers did business, was located directly adjacent to the railroad tracks close to the middle of town. It included an office, two grain elevators, several feed warehouses, a dairy store, and the butcher/meat storage shop. There was always a bustle of activity in the small office

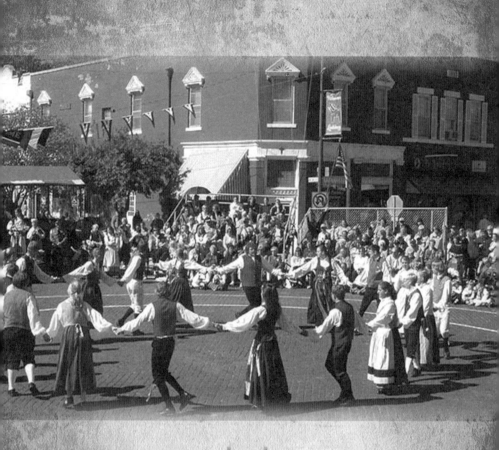

Young folk dancers on the
Main Street of Lindsborg
help celebrate the biennial
October "Svensk Hyllningsfest"
Festival, first organized in 1941,
to honor the community's
Swedish heritage (c2007)

as the farmers exchanged goods, collected receipts for their produce, and paid for purchases.

We brought our wheat, corn, milk, cream and eggs to the Farmers' Union to sell, and we went there to store our butchered meat. It's where we bought our ice, our fertilizer for the wheat fields, and our 100-pound bags of chicken feed and corn meal and other supplements for the animals.

But it was Main Street that gave Lindsborg its charm and character in my day, and that remains true today.

Two blocks to the west of the railroad tracks, Main Street runs north and south, parallel to US 81. It is lined with a variety of cedar, Chinese elm, and oak trees, and it is paved with red bricks for about ten blocks through the center of town. When I was growing up, the bricks gave Lindsborg a quaint appearance and set it apart from the neighboring towns, as did the fact that most of its residential side streets had sidewalks, were paved and had concrete curbs.

There was only one full block of stores and restaurants along Main Street, though there were also a few stores scattered along a second block and just off Main. These included the Post Office and the old Brunswick Hotel, which had already closed when I was a child.

The Farmers State Bank and the Swedish-American Insurance Company anchored the Main Street commercial strip at one end. Although there was another small diner-type restaurant down the block, Pat's Cafe was the primary eating spot. Two drugstores, virtually across the street from each other, served the community. Each had a soda fountain and a few tables where customers could sit while sipping their drinks. There were also a barbershop, a gift shop, a stationery store, the

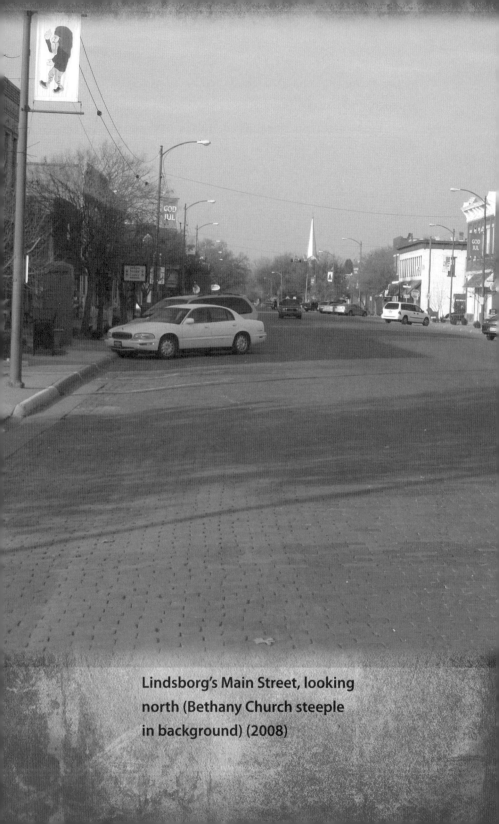

Lindsborg's Main Street, looking
north (Bethany Church steeple
in background) (2008)

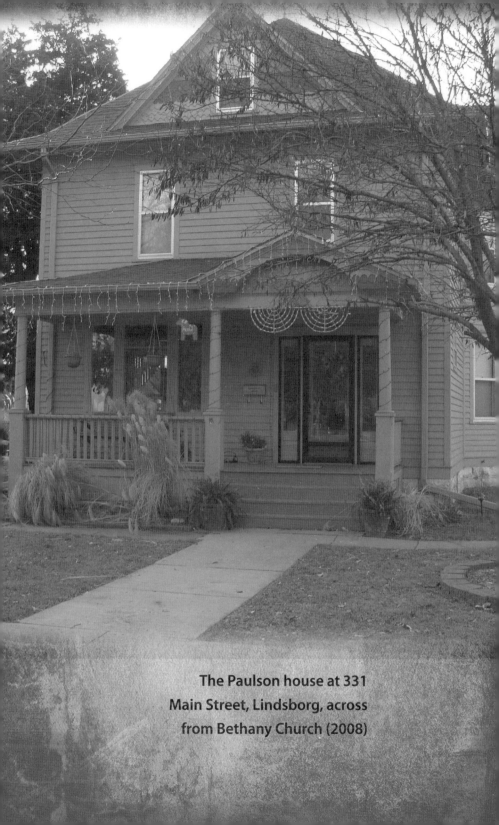

The Paulson house at 331
Main Street, Lindsborg, across
from Bethany Church (2008)

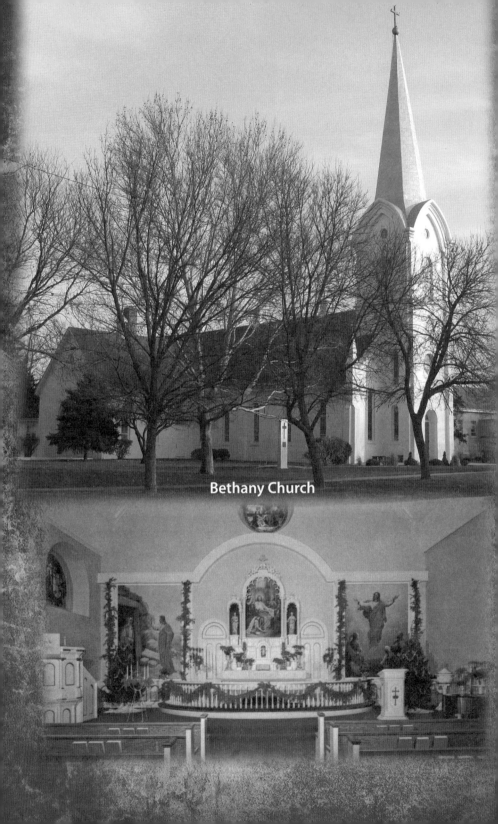

Bethany Church

Gambles' hardware store, the Hansons' men's and boy's shop, a small dress shop, and a grocery store.

Probably the most popular store on Main Street was the bakery-cafe, where two coffee pots were constantly brewing and you poured your cup yourself. There was always a pleasant mix of adults and school-age patrons that included farmers pausing briefly after a trip to the Farmers' Union, salespeople on a coffee break, and teachers and students from the local high school and college having a bite to eat.

Through my high school years, Main Street also boasted a small movie theatre, with a popcorn machine and a soda dispenser. The rows of seats had an aisle on each side. The theatre closed after I graduated from high school and was shuttered for decades. Today it is used for special events such as concerts and community meetings.

My grandparents had moved from the farm to 331 North Main when my father married. The Paulson house was on the far corner of the second block north from the commercial portion of Main Street, directly across the street from Bethany Church and the church parsonage. It was also only half a block from the North Park. The brick portion of Main Street extended past the house, a well-built and well-appointed piece of real estate that was considered prime property in a prime location.

Just a block from my grandparents' home, on the other side of North Park, was Bethany College. Its original building, referred to fondly by Bethany grads as *Old Main*, housed both dormitories and classrooms.

In my day, Lindsborg's Main Street was a beautiful, idyllic setting. It still is.

MILDRED

Of all my friends at the Smoky Hill School, Mildred Nordberg was the one with whom I had the most special relationship. The Nordbergs were tangentially related to our family, since Mildred's mother was a sister of David Hillgren.

I spent a lot of time at the Nordberg farm. It was about two miles from ours, midway between our farm and US 81 and just a few yards off the Roxbury Road to the south. Leroy and Miriam, with much help from their children, Lloyd, Mildred, and Lester, farmed several hundred acres, raised 60 to 80 head of cattle, and ran a substantial dairy operation of probably two dozen Holstein cows.

A half acre had been carved out of one of the Nordberg fields a short distance from the main farmhouse, also alongside the Roxbury Road. There a carefully groomed lawn of buffalo grass surrounded a second, small house, with its own small car garage, a flower garden, and a short, sanded driveway.

From the little front porch of the house you'd enter a little living room and through the back door you'd enter a little kitchen. Upstairs were two little bedrooms. It was like something out of a fairytale book, miniaturized and almost too perfect to be real. But all was not as it seemed.

Leroy Nordberg's sister, Esther lived in the house with their ailing mother, Naomi who suffered from the glandular deficiency that causes the body to store water. As a result, Naomi had become enormously oversized. Sadly, she could not leave the house—or even her chair, not even to sleep—for the last years of her life. On hot summer days, she suffered mightily.

My Mom volunteered Arnold's and my help to weed Esther's flower garden and mow the lawn several times during the summers when I was ten or eleven and he was thirteen or fourteen. Using hand mowers and weeding by hand, we spent all day on the job. For our labors, we were paid 25 cents apiece plus delicious sandwiches and fruit juice for lunch. We did most anything for a meal. The Depression-era song "Brother, Can You Spare a Dime?" could have been our theme song.

We might have been inspired by Leroy's example, for he was an indefatigable worker. I can think of no other farmer in our community who came close to matching Leroy's work ethic. The Nordberg boys, Lloyd and Lester, were respectively five years older and two years younger than I. Farm boys commonly began operating tractors and other farm equipment, even driving pickup trucks, by about age 12, but Lloyd and Lester began at about age 10. Leroy drove them hard to maintain and expand the family's farming operation—much as, I suspect, would have happened in my own house had my father not died.

Mildred Nordberg was a year older than I, and between the ages of 10 and 13, she was the quintessential tomboy. I visited her house every chance I got because Millie was a great playmate.

The Nordbergs' horses included "Billie," a brown-and-white colt mid-size between a Shetland and a normal horse—just right for us. Billie had a gentle disposition, which also was just right, because Millie was something of an acrobat, riding Billie bareback and barefoot standing up! Sometimes we took turns riding him and other times we rode him bareback together.

Millie asked Lloyd to make a trapeze, which he suspended from the very peak of the roof over their barn's hayloft. Then, we'd stack up alfalfa bales at one end of the loft to form a launch platform, and away we'd go! I managed to swing upside down with my knees hooked over the bar. Millie, an acrobat, could hang just by her heels.

The good times with Millie came to an end one day when we were riding Billie, bareback as usual. Something scared the horse. He made a quick sidestep, and we tumbled rather hard to the ground. Although shaken, we were not hurt. The next time I went over to Millie's place, though, she announced that her mother had said bareback riding and trapeze derring-do were no longer a good idea now that Millie was no longer a little girl. I had no idea what she was talking about.

That incident occurred the same year the Smoky Hill School closed and Millie and I began to go to school in Lindsborg. We were placed in different grades. As we made new friends and were no longer together in a single classroom, we drifted apart.

INJUSTICE

Smoky Hill Township School had closed because there weren't enough children to justify the expense of running it. Its former students were driven into Lindsborg, where we joined the town kids and matriculated through high school. For the most part, I had been happy in that one-room schoolhouse, but after an unpleasant experience in my final year I was ready for change.

Pearl Nelson was the teacher when I entered first grade and throughout my second and third years at the school. By all accounts, she was greatly admired by all the parents and our community as a whole.

When I was in grades four and five, and Arnold was completing grades seven and eight, the teacher was Miss Buffington. In the absence of Miss Nelson, our school days proceeded less smoothly. I was too young to create any problems, but Arnold had a mischievous streak and Arlen Patrick, who didn't like to lose, displayed a bit of a temper on the schoolyard. I recall many conversations between Mom and other parents about school issues.

Things between Miss Buffington and me started to turn unpleasant after we went on a school trip, either to see the vast salt mines in Hutchinson or to see the State Juvenile Detention facility, two outings I remember vividly. Four of us were riding in Miss Buffington's car, an old Ford coupe vintage 1937. I was in the back with my good friend Anita Finney and another girl— either Mildred, or Barbara Patrick, or Anita's sister, Rosalie. We were on US Highway 81, still only a two-lane road and unbelievably dangerous by today's standards. A major north-south thoroughfare, it had every kind of traffic—oil tankers, semi-trailer trucks, sand trucks, and so on.

It was after dark—I remember the oncoming headlights— and there was a lot of chatter in the car. We were nearly home when Miss Buffington pulled out of our lane to pass a car, thinking she had sufficient space to move into the oncoming traffic. I happened to look up at the very moment she darted back into our lane, just before an oncoming car whizzed by, horn blaring. We had avoided a collision by only a second or two. Miss Buffington breathed a huge sigh of relief, but the other kids hadn't even noticed.

My trouble with Miss Buffington began the next day. She called my mother and accused me of rifling through her purse on the ride home! I was dumbfounded by this false accusation. I had no idea what she was talking about, and I was innocent. But no one believed me, not even Mom. Though I adamantly denied ever touching the teacher's purse (and no such move could have been further from my mind), Mom insisted that I apologize to Miss Buffington. It was a terrible injustice.

I made the apology with my fingers crossed behind my back, and I hated Miss Buffington from that day forward. It was a blessing to me that Smoky Hill closed its doors the following school year. I was able to make a fresh start in sixth grade in Lindsborg's school system.

GLENN

We had a couple of memorable holiday dinners before my sister Ruth and her husband Glenn moved to Fairbanks, Alaska.

They had decided to explore the larger world, pack their suitcases and head for Fairbanks to take advantage of the Homestead Act of 1946, enacted to encourage the population of that state by giving land grants to settlers.

They were the proverbial match made in heaven. Glenn was tall, dark and handsome, and Ruth, a tall, fair-skinned blonde, cut an equally striking appearance. When she met Glenn, she had been wearing her favorite red dress and a red hat. He had immediately dubbed her "Red" and called her that for the rest of his life.

Raised in Texas, Glenn was an outdoor type of guy, and his addition to our family was a real shot in the arm for us all. He was affable, playful, always upbeat, and just enough older to bring a sense of a man in charge. What's more, he always seemed to enjoy our entire family.

Looking for fun and hoping for a reaction, I would poke Glenn in the stomach or make some wisecrack. To my delight he inevitably responded, *"You're cruisin' for a bruisin'."*

When he married Ruth, Glenn was in the Air Force, stationed at the Smoky Hill Air Force Base just south of Salina. They initially moved to a basement apartment in Salina and then to a small house in Lindsborg, so we saw them a lot. Glenn frequently commented on the fact that whenever Johnny, Arnold or I passed the refrigerator we'd open the door and look inside for something to snack on. "Don't you kids ever stop eating?" he'd ask.

Glenn loved a good joke, and he pulled a memorable one after the last Thanksgiving dinner at his and Ruth's house. She had prepared an enormous smorgasbord with turkey, stuffing, ham, sweet potatoes topped with melted marshmallows, mashed potatoes, carrots, string beans, broccoli and asparagus. Then came the desserts—apple pie, pumpkin pie and Ruth's special chocolate cake.

When the marathon eating was finally over, Glenn seized his moment. "Are you guys full?" he asked, with a twinkle in his eye. "Sure you don't want another slice of ham? How about another piece of pie?" We all just groaned.

"I want to be sure you're not hungry," he continued. "And I think you can eat more." With that, he pulled out half a dozen of the giant-sized Hershey chocolate bars that cost 25 cents back then.

"Come on, fellas, you can't go home hungry!" As we held our stomachs and groaned some more, Glenn just laughed and laughed.

Glenn left his most lasting impression on me a month later, on Christmas Day, right before he and Ruth were due to leave town. We had finished our early afternoon dinner, the dishes

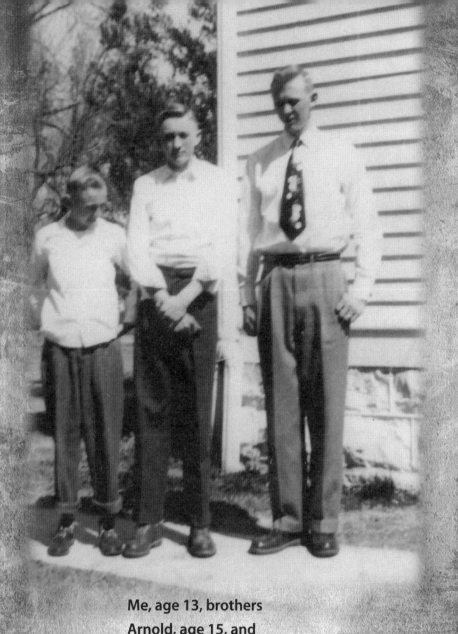

Me, age 13, brothers
Arnold, age 15, and
Johnny, age 20 at
the backdoor of
grandparents' house in
Lindsborg (Easter 1951)

were sitting around the end of the dining room table, close to the kitchen.

I was in the kitchen, where Johnny was showing Glenn a shotgun a neighbor had lent him for pheasant hunting. It was a single barrel, 16-gauge gun with a beautifully polished wood butt. When Johnny started to demonstrate the loading and trigger mechanisms, he was holding the gun horizontally, its barrel pointed toward the dining room.

Glenn put his hand on the gun barrel and gently pushed it down, saying, "You should always point the barrel of a gun down whenever you're handling it." At that very instant, *KER-BLAM*! The gun went off, blowing an inch-wide hole in our kitchen floor just six inches from my foot!

At first, nobody moved. We were thunderstruck, our faces drained ghost-white. Then, it was bedlam. Everyone was shouting at Johnny: "What the hell!" "Christ Almighty!" "How could you not know the gun was loaded?" Glenn was silent, thinking only of the staggering potential tragedy that had been avoided. Mom, and possibly both sisters too, would surely have been killed.

My lifelong distaste for guns or hunting of any sort dates from this incident.

CHRISTMAS

No matter how little money we had, Christmas was a special time in my childhood. There was always a tree to decorate, a pile of presents to open and lots of food, including candy and nuts, to eat over the holiday break from school.

Weeks in advance, Mom would bake dozens of cookies,

mostly gingersnaps, peanut butter and shortbread.

Then she'd buy dried lutefisk imported from Sweden by our local grocery store. Mom would soak it in water for three or four days before she cooked it. A white meat fish, fairly light and flakey, it's rather bland. So Mom would enliven the taste by making up a tiny jar of hot—very hot—mustard from a powder base. Actually, *very hot* is an understatement. Only a dab of that mustard would have you grabbing for the water glass.

She also prepared a large baked ham with a honey and cinnamon glaze. It was spiced with cloves, and I was the one who'd stick them into the glazed surface. The ham was big enough to last several days and then the bone went into a split-pea soup. Mom used foodstuffs very efficiently!

Naturally, we also had sweet potatoes with marshmallow topping, mashed potatoes with brown gravy, and a variety of vegetables.

We opened our presents on Christmas Eve. We'd go to dinner in Lindsborg at Aunt Helga's, always starting with a round of glogg, the famous Swedish drink, made of warmed, spiced and sweetened wine. She went all out for us, but we preferred the meal that would be prepared by Mom the next day. After eating, we opened presents at our grandparents' house, and then we rushed home to open everything under our own tree. It was always a late night, so we boys slept in on Christmas morning while Mom made the final preparations for our early afternoon dinner.

Our church celebrated the holiday with a service on Christmas morning—at 6 a.m. I'm afraid we usually missed it, but for a couple of years during my high school days, I not only made the service but also played my trombone with a brass quartet in the belfry to call the worshippers to the church. It was ridiculously early, the temperature was freezing or below, our hands, lips and instruments were all cold as ice and we were sitting in a drafty, tiny room 30 or 40 feet high. It's amazing what kids will do for their superiors.

I can still see the blue lips of our trumpet player, Robert Leaf, as he struggled to purse them against the cold mouthpiece of his horn. But, being kids, we had a big chuckle afterwards when we thought how poorly we had played under such duress. Naturally, however, the congregation loved the music. If only they had known!

FRAUD

As if Mom hadn't had enough to swallow as a result of my father's death, she was dealt a second blow when my grandfather died in 1949, ten years later, at age ninety-five. He was ill for several years beforehand, and my only memory of him is of his lying in bed.

For as long as I can remember, my father's sister Helga lived with my grandparents in the Lindsborg house and cared for them in their declining years. Helga had married and had two sons, Hilding and Carl Helge. But her husband deserted her—he simply walked out the front door of their house one morning without a word and was never heard from again—and she was forced to take her young children and move into my grandparents' house. There she remained for the rest of her life.

My father and grandfather had made an arrangement. My father paid for the house in Lindsborg for my grandparents so he could raise his own family on the farm, and in return, my grandfather had made a will that left the original farm of 320 acres, the farmhouse, and all the farm buildings and machinery to my father.

But when my grandfather's will was read, there was a codicil—an amendment. Helga, their caretaker, was given the house in Lindsborg—PLUS 160 acres of our farm! Signe, another sister, was bequeathed the separate 80-acre field. No share was bequeathed to a third sister, Agnes, who had predeceased my father and had no heirs.

Not until I was in college did I learn from one of my brothers that the signature on the codicil to my grandfather's will was shaky and virtually illegible—the sort one would expect to see if one person was guiding the hand of another person holding the pen. Who but Helga was living in the house while my grandfather was in poor health and dying? Who but Helga would benefit from a major change in the original provisions of the will—a change that was greatly detrimental to my mother? Who but Helga would have been the guiding hand?

Still later, in law school, I read numerous cases where the caretaker of a sick or dying person drew up a codicil to that person's will, changing its provisions in his or her favor. The courts routinely threw these out, usually finding undue influence or outright fraud on the part of the caretaker or finding the deceased to have been mentally incompetent at the time the codicil was made. I immediately realized that my grandfather's codicil was a classic example of this sort. If challenged, the codicil would never have been upheld in court.

What a dastardly deed—stealing half of the farm my father had worked to build up for nearly forty years, knowing that my mother and her young boys had been struggling to make ends meet ever since his death. Helga had made that struggle even more onerous by refusing to allow my grandfather to pay any part of my father's medical expenses which forced my mother to take out a mortgage on the farm that took years to pay off.

Unrepentant and unashamed, Helga continued to live in my grandparents' very comfortable home in Lindsborg, thanks to my father, and maintained a holier-than-thou attitude, presenting herself as a pious, church-going pillar of the community. What audacity! Inexplicably, she outlived virtually everyone, dying finally at one hundred and three. I can only hope she got her just desserts in Hell!

When I learned in law school of the terrible injustice foisted upon my mother (far too late to do anything about it), I was astonished that Helga had gotten away with such a patently unfair and obvious deception, and, moreover, that no one in the community had come to my mother's aid. I confronted Mom with my newfound knowledge, but she said only, "What could I do? I had to live where I was. I thought I couldn't remain there if I made an enemy of Helga."

Looking back, I admire my mother's strength of character. Despite all the odds and Helga's evil hand in depleting my mother's property and her income—when wheat-growing land is rented, one-third of the income goes to the landowner and two-thirds to the renting farmer—Mom kept us together on the farm throughout all our school years.

At the time of my grandfather's death, Johnny had already shown he was capable of running the whole show at just age 19. However, Helga's greed reduced our farmland to only 160 acres. Taking into account the pastureland on our farm and space for our cattle and pigs, we only had some 120 acres for crops. That put a huge damper on Johnny's ability to make a good living off the remaining farmland. He did, however, keep us afloat. And that was quite an accomplishment.

PICNICS

Despite Aunt Helga's disgraceful behavior, our ability to enjoy ourselves continued unabated.

Among the most popular entertainments of my childhood were summer picnics, which were usually held in one of Lindsborg's two town parks.

The North Park, near my grandparents' home, was notable for its Swensson Memorial Band Shell, a small goldfish pond and an equally small wading pool that was no more than perhaps 30" deep at one end.

The Bethany Church always held an early summer picnic for the Sunday school classes in the North Park, and I remember hanging on the fence surrounding the pool and watching the goldfish for endless amounts of time. On rare occasions, Arnold and I even put on swimsuits and splashed around in the baby pool.

The South Park, adjacent to the Smoky River on the south border of Lindsborg, was our preferred picnic location when I was little because it was slightly bigger and a bit shadier than the North Park. It also offered a pair of concrete tennis courts and horseshoe pits as well as swings and teeter-totters for the little ones. By the time I was 13 or 14, Lindsborg had built a new pool there, and South Park had become everyone's preferred picnic site.

Each of Mom's ladies' clubs sponsored an annual picnic, as did the church and our 4-H club. No doubt there were others I didn't know of or can't recall.

The food was always the same, yet I never had enough of it. There was fried spring chicken, potato salad, Jell-O filled with diced fruit, peas and carrots, and string beans, all freshly prepared and toted by the mothers.

But the biggest treat was the ice cream. It always came from Bachman's, our local dairy store, in large 3- or 4-gallon containers wrapped in a heavy, thick canvas bag. One man scooped it out and filled up cone after cone—as many as you could eat! And how delicious it was! Even in New York City, only the ice cream produced by the Sedutto family of Staten Island compares favorably with Bachman's of Lindsborg in the 1950s.

My neighbor Clarence Esping loved to ask, "Do you eat to live, or do you live to eat?" That question genuinely stumped me—particularly if I were savoring the memory of those picnics. I have never forgotten how much pleasure those glorious Sunday afternoon events brought me.

SCANDAL

Although my mother squelched the potential scandal involving Helga's fraudulent manipulation of my grandfather's will, like residents of small towns everywhere, people were generally subject to close scrutiny. So it was stunning to learn that another supposedly upstanding citizen had broken the law in several ways.

Lindsborg was a religious community. Although there were fewer than 3000 townspeople, Lindsborg in the 1940s and

50s supported five congregations: Bethany Lutheran, Messiah Lutheran, a Methodist church, a Baptist church, and a Mission Friends congregation. Our family belonged to Bethany, whose congregation of 400 members was the largest. The treasurer of the church was Carl Hanson, who with his equally well-regarded brother owned Hanson Clothiers on Main Street.

The town was dry. The closest source for alcoholic drinks was nine miles away, in Marquette, a tiny one-horse town with perhaps a half-dozen stores. In my early teens, we got news of an automobile accident on the road to Marquette. A car driven by a high school senior had crashed head-on into a small bridge abutment. The driver and another student were not seriously injured, but a third passenger, Carl Hanson, was instantly killed. The group had no doubt been on a beer run. That alone embarrassed the family.

But more embarrassing news came to light when Carl's estate was reviewed. It turned out that he had embezzled more than $100,000 from the Bethany Church treasury.

JOY RIDES

Farm boys and girls typically started operating farm equipment, including cars and trucks, at age twelve. At 13, we were given provisional drivers licenses, which permitted us to drive alone so long as we were going directly to and from a predetermined destination approved by a parent. You can just imagine how closely that restriction was followed.

I started to drive our old 1937 Plymouth pickup truck at age 12, in the middle of a wheat field (thank goodness). Johnny was my self-appointed instructor, though he wouldn't have been my choice for the role. He was hardly a model of patience.

As you may know, learning the proper timing for the use of the clutch and gas pedal is like learning to ride a bike—impossible until suddenly you get the hang of it, and then it's as if you had been doing it forever. After killing the engine eight or ten times, I finally got going in the wheat field without burning out the clutch. Miracles never cease!

When I was 13, my Saturday mornings were taken up with Catechism study at the church. That was the perfect excuse to hop in the car alone and drive into town. I had the pickup. Everyone else had some version of his or her parents' cars. After class we'd have a *wild and crazy time*—essentially a group joyride. Piling into two or three vehicles, we all just drove around, following each other. None of us was too sure of himself, and we all drove much too fast for our handling abilities.

A favorite destination for our Saturday morning tomfoolery was Coronado Heights, a 400-to-500-foot-high mound just three or four miles northwest of Lindsborg. Local lore has it that the Spanish explorer Coronado visited the site in 1541 in his quest for gold. A fort-like sandstone building sits at the top of Coronado Heights, and there are several stone and concrete tables for picnicking. The road circling the mound to the top was poorly maintained, but the trip was worthwhile for the 360-degree vista of the entire Smoky Valley.

On one of our Height excursions, a classmate driver just ahead of me misjudged his speed coming down the mound. He failed to make the last turn at the bottom and his car caromed into the ditch, finally shaking to a stop. Pushing and pulling, we managed to get the car out.

No one was hurt, but it was a sobering experience for a lot of very young people.

BLACKIE

My adventures with Blackie taught me to be careful of what you wish for. You just might get it.

A small rodeo, sponsored by the 4-H organization, was held at an arena about 18 miles south of our farm near McPherson.

I'm not sure why I was even at the rodeo, or how it was that Johnny was there, too. Certainly we weren't traveling in the same circles, since he was 20 and I was only fourteen. I was wandering around in the crowd with some other kids when someone shouted, "Hey, kids, come get your ropes and try catching a calf!"

Some of the cattle farmers in the area had each donated a yearling steer, and a contest had been arranged. All the kids would be given a lariat. First the young steers would be let loose in the arena, and then the kids would be let loose in the arena to try to lasso one of them. Whoever caught a calf could keep it provided he or she agreed to raise and feed the calf until it could be exhibited at the County Fair the following year.

Everybody took off toward the contest, and I didn't want to be left behind, so I ran with the group. In a moment, I had my rope and was standing in a crowd of boys and a smaller number of girls. At the far end of the arena, I could see perhaps a dozen calves, milling about anxiously.

"OK, kids, GO!" It was bedlam. A gate opened and everyone took off — a herd of shouting, running kids, all trying to be first to get to the calves! Naturally, the calves were terrified. As we caught up to them, they ran right past us, thundering to the opposite end. Rats!

All the kids turned to race back, but in the confusion, I was knocked to the ground and left momentarily alone. Just as

I got up and started to follow the others, a nearby rodeo clown came close.

"Kid," he said quietly, "Don't go anywhere. They're just gonna chase the calves right back here! Just wait!"

Sure enough, here came the calves, all the kids in hot pursuit. I wasn't exactly comfortable with a few hundred pounds of beef hurtling right down on the clown and me. I closed my eyes almost completely, but I stuck out my loop of rope and bravely held my ground. Amazingly, one of the calves ran right through my loop. I had actually roped a calf! WOW!

Johnny was less than thrilled with my win. "You're going to feed and take care of that for a year? Who's buying the feed? How're we getting him home?"

The next day was better. Johnny got a neighbor's trailer and we drove back to the arena, loaded up Blackie, and headed for home.

Blackie was a thoroughbred Black Angus steer about a year old and weighing 80 or 90 pounds. I cared for that calf for the next year, feeding it corn meal and extra food supplements along with alfalfa hay, cane stalk, and grass. But there were problems.

For one thing, Blackie just never seemed to have much appetite. I almost always found food left in his feeding trough. Though I'd empty it and replace it with fresh meals, I did so to no avail. Also, Blackie had a wild streak that I couldn't break. This was especially frustrating since I was required to show Blackie at the next year's county fair—to lead him with a halter, walking in a circle in front of the judge, then bring him to attention, with his front and back legs aligned. I worked endlessly with Blackie on his deportment, but he had an independent spirit.

Arriving at the county fair with Blackie a year later was a real eye-opener. I was astonished at the size of the other steers that had been caught at the arena. By comparison, Blackie was a midget.

Eventually we were in the ring, waiting for the judge's decision on my performance and on Blackie's development. I will never forget the judge's booming voice, as he placed a white ribbon—last place—on Blackie, "Looks like this young feller got tired of carryin' thuh feed bucket!" the judge added sarcastically. I should have been mortified. Instead, I was simply relieved that I had gotten Blackie to walk and stand reasonably still in the arena without running away!

I sold Blackie right after the fair and bought a bicycle.

LIFE LESSONS

The hardest part of making the transition in sixth grade from the Smoky Hill country school to public school in Lindsborg was having to eat in the schoolroom while most of the kids, who lived nearby, went home for lunch. Otherwise, the move wasn't difficult. I felt comfortable in my new school and learned a couple of important life lessons during junior high.

I had already known several of my new classmates from our church, and on the first or second day, something happened that helped me establish a good reputation with all of them. I had been assigned a desk somewhere in the middle of an outside row. Shortly after the class came to attention and the teacher began discussing the day's topic, a mouse appeared near the front of the room. The teacher let out a soft shriek and started to climb onto her chair. Half my classmates drew up their legs, and more shrieks rang out.

At that moment the mouse turned and began to run along the wall near my desk and in my direction. Instinctively, I jumped out of my seat and ran toward the wall, thinking, I suppose, to trap it. I jammed my foot against the wall. To my surprise, I crushed the mouse dead under my shoe! I picked it up by its tail to the cheers of the class, and the teacher let out a sigh of relief. Bobby Paulson was a person no mouse should mess with!

But for a boy to really establish himself in Lindsborg, as I suspect is the case in all small towns, you had to play on the football team, or you became a target for all sorts of taunts and innuendos, none pleasant. Fortunately, that wasn't a problem.

By the time I entered junior high, Eskil Anderson, an English teacher fresh out of college who was something of an athlete, had formed a team of seventh- and eighth-graders and lobbied for uniforms. As our coach, he inspired all of us with his enthusiasm, and I learned much of the game's strategy from him. Frankly, I don't remember if we even played in competition with schools from surrounding towns, but all in all, the boys had great fun.

Eager and energetic, easy to approach, the teacher made me feel very comfortable in his presence—perhaps too comfortable. Seeing him on Main Street one day, I greeted him casually. "Hi Eskil. How's it going? "

"Bob, you need to call me Mr. Anderson," he said. "I'm still your teacher." Lesson one.

Our eighth grade teacher, Ruthie Asche, was a bit eccentric but obviously loved her job. She did everything with a flourish—and that extended even to her handwriting. Into every capital letter she inserted a curlicue or added a final twirl. I liked her style, but then I discovered in the schoolyard that I had acquired the unfortunate reputation of being a teacher's pet. So I stopped volunteering information in the class. Lesson two.

CRASH

Having started plowing with a tractor at 12 or 13, by age 14 I had had quite a bit of experience—though not enough, it turned out.

We owned two tractors. One was a huge, lumbering John Deere D-model whose front and back wheels were widely spaced. The other was a lighter and easier-to-manipulate Allis-Chalmers. It was designed like a tricycle, with two large back wheels and two small front wheels close together.

The John Deere was so big it didn't even have brakes. It stopped when you disengaged the clutch by pulling on a long lever right next to the steering wheel.

The Allis-Chalmers had a foot clutch much like that of a car. However, I could engage it only by sliding forward in the seat while simultaneously pulling back on the steering wheel to gain leverage for my leg, which had to be fully extended. The Allis had brake levers for each back wheel. By braking one back wheel as the front wheels were turned, you could make very sharp turns.

The Deere, which had only one forward gear, was easier to drive because the right front wheel could run in the furrow made by the last plowing. Letting the wheel be guided by the sidewall of the furrow, I could manipulate the plow levers without stopping by twisting my upper body around, leaning back, and stretching one arm to reach the forward end of the lever to raise or lower the depth of the plowshares.

The Allis had a four-speed gearshift that you had to change frequently, depending on the *pull* or *drag* of the plow. That in turn depended on the depth at which the plowshares were set or the type of soil being plowed, which often changed over a quarter or half-mile stretch. Twisting and leaning back to reach the levers of the plow while keeping the Allis on a straight line without having the furrow as a guide was a challenge.

At each end of the field, you had to *trip up* the plow—pull the plowshares out of the ground—and simultaneously turn the tractor and drive to the next furrow. Once the tractor and plow were aligned in the next furrow, the plow was *tripped down*, and the plowshares were dropped to whatever depth was set by the levers. The practice of *tripping* also involved reaching back and pulling on a trip cord that released or engaged a ratchet-and-pawl type of mechanism.

The day of our great adventure, 17-year-old Arnold and I were plowing an 80-acre tract of our wheat fields. We were at the point where all the soil was turned over on each side and only a sliver of land was left in between. Plowing that sliver creates a *dead furrow*, a little trough, the whole length of the field.

I was plowing the dead furrow going north, while Arnold was plowing the same dead furrow headed south. I was assuming Arnold would trip up and pull out. And Arnold was expecting me to do the same.

We were heading right for each other. When I realized Arnold had no intention of yielding, I grabbed the clutch lever, hoping to stop the contraption. To my horror, the lever stuck. I threw my full weight behind it to no avail.

Smack dab in the middle of an 80-acre field, SMASH—a

head-on collision!

There was much yelling, screaming and confusion in the aftermath. I don't remember if I did get the Deere out of gear, nor do I recall if Arnold ever stopped the Allis. The crankshaft protruding from the front of the Allis punched a hole through the radiator of the Deere, leaving it out of commission for several weeks. Neither of us was hurt—not that anyone asked. The cost for repairs was several hundred dollars. That was the hardest to swallow.

As usual, poor Arnold, as the older one, got the brunt of the blame. Of course, Johnny was enraged, Mom grew another set of grey hairs, and Arnold and I had to hide our sheepish faces for weeks on end.

NEAR MISSES

The tractor crash wasn't the first vehicular misadventure the Paulson boys had had. Nor would it be the last.

When I was 10 or 11, I was riding with Paul on US 81, not far from Lindsborg. He was at the wheel of the car, a four-door relic whose back doors opened at the center post. His wife, Emma, was in the front seat with JoAnn, then a baby. I was in back with my mother and Arnold, and Paul and Emma's three-year-old, Darrell, was standing between my knees. As Emma later recalled, Paul was speeding along, so as a cautionary measure, she called to me over her shoulder.

"Bobby, would you lock the back door? Just push down on that little thing on the top."

The next few seconds were terrifying. Rather than push down on the locking peg by the windowsill, I pushed down on the door handle. The oncoming rush of wind made the door fly open, and Darrell was immediately sucked out of the car. Fortunately, I was holding onto one of his hands. For a split second, I was leaning halfway out of the door, still holding his hand, and I watched as his legs bounced back and forth, coming so close to the back wheel I was afraid they might get caught under it. Paul immediately pulled over close to the edge of the pavement, so Darrell was bouncing on grass and dirt, which were relatively soft as it was raining at the time.

I had a horrible decision to make: Should I hang on and risk Darrell's bouncing under the rear wheel, or let go, so he would fall onto the soft shoulder of the road? I let go when I saw his legs bounce away from the car. Naturally, I hadn't anticipated that Darrell's eyebrow would be caught on the bottom edge of the door. He suffered a slash from the top of one eyebrow to the middle of his forehead.

By the time Paul stopped the car, Darrell was already up and running towards us, screaming, blood streaming down his face. It was a terrible outcome, but could have been worse. We drove directly to the office of Dr. Holwerda, who patched up Darrell's forehead and assured us he would be fine. Darrell did recover quickly. Unfortunately, there was little knowledge of or access to plastic surgery in those days, at least not in our area. Today, they'd deal with such a cut so it would hardly be noticeable, but Darrell was left with a permanent scar from the wound.

Several years later, after Johnny came home from Korea unscathed—he had been assigned to heavy equipment operation and for the most part ran a bulldozer to build roads—he was in a bad auto accident while coming home from army camp on a furlough. He and two other draftees were in the back seat of the car when it plowed into the rear of a semi-trailer truck that had stopped on the road in a driving rainstorm. The boys were thrown forward with such impact that their knees punched six holes into the back of the front seat. Although John was found wandering in a field after the accident, suffering from shock, he had no broken bones and was released from the hospital after a few days.

On another occasion, Arnold was driving—*drag racing, most likely!*—our pickup, the '37 Plymouth, when he rolled it over. The incident occurred somewhere near Marquette. The location tells it all! Marquette was the nearest town that sold beer.

Looking back, I think this incident was an example of Arnold's reaction to what he experienced as John's tyranny by cutting loose from time to time. As the *de facto* manager of the farm, Johnny was a very effective, but very tough, boss, and he was particularly hard on Arnold, who he said was "too smart for his own good" *Devil-may-care by nature*, Arnold was at the time in his late teens, when most kids chafe under authority.

Although both Arnold and the truck suffered only a few scratches, Johnny went crazy, fists flying. Mom intervened, saving the day for Arnold.

Later on, working the winter season as an apprentice carpenter, building *cookie-cutter* houses that were part of the post-War housing boom, Arnold put aside enough money to buy his own car, a 1946 Buick Roadmaster. It was a heavy, four-door model, with a huge front hood housing a large V-8 engine. (In those days, gas consumption was not an issue.) He and Raymond Finney drove it to Tucson after high school graduation.

A year later, back home, he went on a night of boozing and fell asleep at the wheel. Though he totaled the car against a telephone pole, he was unhurt because the size of the car protected him. Another near tragedy averted.

CHORES

We may have had our occasional misadventures, but doing farm work developed not only physical strength but also mental grit.

My mother remembered when times were even harder. Prior to the development of combines, my grandfather, and also my father, used mules to pull the plows, disks, and harrows, then used a machine called a binder to cut and tie the ripe wheat into bundles. The bundles were stacked into separate little tepee-shaped *shocks* in the field and eventually fed into a thresher that separated the wheat kernels from the stalks.

Threshing crews of 15 to 18 men followed the harvest season, moving north from Texas to the Dakotas, and from farm to farm, to pick up the wheat bundles, feed them into the thresher and transport the wheat grain to the storage elevator for sale.

Throughout the seven to ten days of the harvest, Mom was expected to bring a noontime lunch for the crew out to the field, return with afternoon coffee and cake, and finally prepare an evening dinner meal at the end of the workday for the entire crew as well as her own family of seven children.

Even with the newer machinery, during my high school years we had plenty of back-breaking work. When harvesting wheat, for example, we always saved about 200 bushels for seeding for the following year. That meant transferring several loads of wheat kernels from the pickup truck into a grain bin, tossing it a shovelful at a time six feet or more. As the truckload diminished, the throwing distance increased. Just standing in the wheat grain was a challenge. The loose kernels made your footing unsteady, and you might sink in up to your ankles. With the temperature often in the high nineties, the sweat and dust were stifling.

Bringing in the alfalfa hay was doubly hard. After the crop was cut and raked into rows, we pitch-forked the alfalfa onto the hayrack in the field and then positioned the hayrack below the door to the barn hayloft. We pitched up the hay, carried it to the back of the hayloft, and did more pitchfork throwing to pile it as high as possible. To harvest and store one crop of alfalfa would take a dozen or more hayrack loads. On occasion, one of our neighbors would bale the alfalfa for us, but that didn't reduce the work much. Each bale weighed 60 to 80 pounds and had to be heaved or hoisted up to the hay wagon and from there to the hayloft. To think of it now—Oohh, my aching back!

One summer, when I was about 13 or 14, our youthful exuberance nearly cost us our hay barn. Johnny, Arnold and I had finished loading the loose alfalfa hay into the hayloft. Since we'd had a good crop, the hayloft was stacked high. So Arnold and I had the bright idea to climb up as high as possible in the rafters and jump onto the stack of alfalfa. We did this for only a half hour or so and then left to finish chores.

The next day, I returned to the hayloft and started to lift some of the hay to feed our cows. I was startled to see smoke rising between the alfalfa leaves. I ran to get help and we boys began feverishly shifting the hay across the hayloft.

What happened was that by jumping on the hay, we had

packed it down, and the combination of heat and moisture in the freshly cut alfalfa set the stage for spontaneous combustion. It was a very close call.

Hoeing our gardens and the potato plants was yet another exhausting exercise, and of course there was all the daily work involved in milking our cows and feeding the pigs. It wasn't just time-consuming. It also required a lot of heavy lifting—lugging 100-pound sacks of feed, hauling and hoisting buckets of slurry and water.

Even filling our gas barrels was a struggle. Our two 50-gallon barrels had to be wrestled from the pickup onto a platform about three feet high, then maneuvered into position and tipped onto their side, with the spigot overhanging the platform. Maneuvering the filled barrels of gas meant tipping them slightly and rolling them on the bottom edge side to side just a few inches at a time and making sure to keep our toes out from under the barrel. You've heard the expression *barrels of fun*? Well, this wasn't.

TREATS

When I was growing up, there wasn't much difference between our lifestyle and that of the upper-class Lindsborg residents. Life was simpler. There weren't many temptations in our local stores—or even in the larger towns nearby.

And while we had a constant struggle to make ends meet, I felt connected to a more comfortable life through the house in Lindsborg even though as a child I didn't know that my father had paid for it. The house was comparable to or better than the other homes in town, with the exception of the residence of the

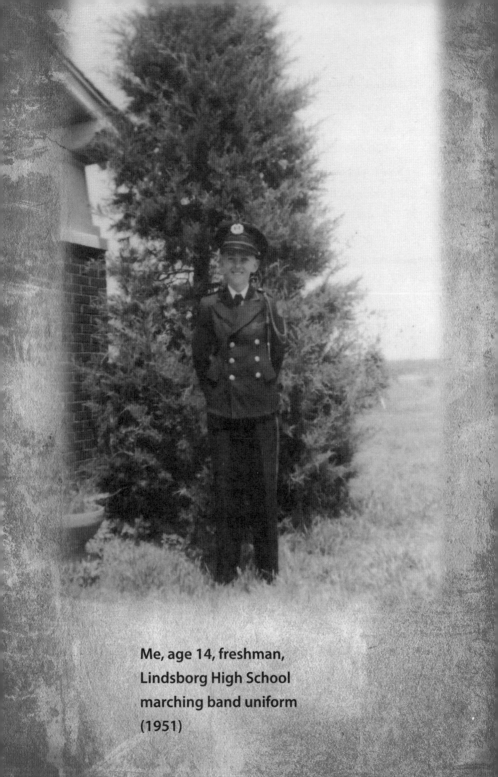

Me, age 14, freshman,
Lindsborg High School
marching band uniform
(1951)

town doctor, William Holwerda.

Shortly after I entered the Lindsborg school system, the Holwerdas purchased a large, rundown house some two miles outside Lindsborg and undertook a massive renovation. Our classmate, Jim Holwerda, invited several schoolmates and me there for a birthday party. The rooms were spacious, the bedrooms were numerous, and the kitchen contained all the latest appliances. For me, the home was an astonishing glimpse into how *the other half* lived.

We were quite satisfied with modest treats like the shopping trip we traditionally made in late August, right before the Smoky Hill School reopened in the fall. In those days, the large chain stores were in Salina, which with its population of 20,000 was almost seven times as big as Lindsborg. We'd sometimes go there to shop at Sears for small tools and appliances or, as a last resort, Montgomery Ward's, since Mom didn't like its merchandise as much.

But for our pre-school needs, we could find what we wanted in McPherson, a town of about 10,000. We'd browse in the bookstore for an hour or more, picking out our new schoolbooks, tablets, workbooks, pencils and other accessories. I don't remember Mom having a list of materials, but somehow she knew what to get for us.

For new school clothes and shoes, we shopped in the McPherson Penny's. Though the Hanson store in Lindsborg sold men's and boy's clothing, we shopped there only in an emergency, since the selection was limited.

As a youngster, I wore high-topped work shoes, similar to hiking boots, white Hanes' briefs, t-shirts, flannel plaid shirts, and blue-and-white striped bib overalls. By the time I entered the Lindsborg school system, I was still wearing bib overalls until I grew out of them, but exclusively as work clothes on the farm. I wouldn't dream of wearing them in public.

For school or other trips into town, only blue jeans would do. Jeans were what everybody wore, and peer pressure ruled, even back then and even in Kansas. When it comes to fashion, there is nothing new under the sun. During one period in high school, some of my friends and I pushed our belts low on our hips and turned up the collars of our shirts. (And New York kids think they are so hip!)

Though we never ate in either of the Lindsborg restaurants as a family, I often enjoyed a hamburger or two with greasy French fries or a root beer float with school chums at one of the drugstores on Main Street.

And when I was a pre-teen, Saturday afternoon at the movies was a special treat. For the astounding price of 12 cents (later jacked up to 25!) we saw a serial segment, a cartoon and a cowboy movie. The serials were especially exciting. At the end of each segment, the hero would be left in some terrible plight. The following week, they'd replay the last scene and—lo and behold!—he would narrowly escape what had appeared to be certain death.

FOOTBALL HERO

Junior high school football was fun, but playing football on the Vikings team during my freshman year in high school was another story.

First, the reader needs to know that I weighed, at most, perhaps 80 pounds at the time. At age 14, I had not yet gotten my teenage growth spurt, so I was only about 5' 6". I've never had a large head, and at the time my head size was probably a size six-and-a-half. Despite these handicaps, or because of them, I was fast and rarely could be outrun, except by my Smoky Hill classmate Lola Hanson, who truly ran like the wind; I never knew anyone faster, boy or girl.

But the football equipment was the sticky part. It was old, beat-up and heavy beyond belief. There were thigh pads, hip pads, rib pads and shoulder pads, all made from a kind of Bakelite plastic and cotton padding. The pants were thick canvas. I borrowed a pair of football shoes— high-topped leather, a size too big, with cone-shaped cleats about 3/4" long. But for me the ultimate insult was the helmet. All of the available helmets for the team were kept in a big box. It was first come, first served. Unfortunately, there was only one helmet under size seven and Jerry Plotner, a sophomore, beat me to it.

I must have been a ridiculous sight. Weighed down by pounds of padding, shoes the weight of those of a deep-sea diver, and a helmet that spun on my head, I was no longer a speed threat. In fact, I couldn't even do some of the warm-up calisthenics. For one, we were told to lie on our backs, hold our hips up with our hands, and scissor-kick our legs back over our heads with the toe of each foot alternately touching the ground. This was impossible for me. My hip pads were so stiff and oversized that my legs couldn't move past a horizontal position.

Naturally, with all these impediments, I never got past the B team in high school. We did, however, play against the B teams of surrounding schools. I have vivid memories of three games in particular.

In those days, there was no such thing as a facemask.

The helmet was Knut Rockneish, cotton padding under a stiff leather wrap, with ineffective canvas support webbing inside. In one game, I was on the punt-receiving team and, lo and behold, the ball was coming straight to me! As I was looking up, watching the ball, I could hear the thundering boots of the opposing team about to bear down. With no choice but to grit my teeth and spin my helmet out of the way (there was no such thing as a "free catch"), I caught the ball and was immediately overwhelmed by a half dozen zealots from the other team.

In another game, I was lined up on offense in the end position—at my fly weight, no other position was conceivable—and ready to run a pass route. As the ball was snapped, my defender coolly rolled his hand into a fist and blind-sided me with an uppercut to my nose! I think that was the defining moment when I knew football was not the game for me.

But I did have a great football moment. It came in a game when I was on the kick-off team shortly before half time. The receiver had the ball and I was tearing down the field. (That may be an overstatement.) Suddenly, all my teammates seem to have disappeared and only the receiver and I were left standing. As we both rushed to a head-on collision, I lowered my head and hit the guy with all my might, shoulder planted into his thighs and my arms wrapped around his knees. He dropped like a rock. A roar came up from my teammates. I was stunned from the impact but tried not to show it. In the locker room, the coach was ecstatic. "If anyone wants to know how to make a tackle, just ask Bobby. That was the best I've seen this year!"

And that was my football career, over at age fourteen. You might think I cleverly ended it on a high note. In fact, an opportunity came my way that left me no choice but to quit the team.

AMAHL AND THE NIGHT VISITORS

I was in the wheat field driving a tractor pulling a plow, wearing a *scuddy* old cap, ears and face covered with dust, when a senior at Bethany College sought me out and offered me the culminating experience in my career as a boy soprano. It was 1952, and I had just turned fifteen.

For as long as I can remember, I had loved to sing. First, I'd sing along with the radio on a long car ride. Then, I would sit on the piano bench next to my sister Ruth and sing as she played. I wonder now how or when she learned, since no one else in the family played the piano.

At 9, I sang my first solo, "Away in a Manger," in a Christmas program presented by our church in Lindsborg. The next year, I began piano lessons in Lindsborg. Each Saturday morning, we brought two or three dozen fresh eggs and perhaps a gallon or two of cream to the Farmers' Union to sell. From the eight to twelve dollars in receipts, Mom would pull a dollar to pay Mrs. Boettcher., who taught me until I was sixteen. I learned to read music with some degree of proficiency, at least well enough to accompany myself in vocal practice. Those dollar lessons would prove invaluable, not only in learning the Amahl role but in allowing me to enjoy my lifetime hobby of singing. (Thank you, Mom!)

As I became able to play a range of music on the piano, Mom often would listen intently while she rocked quietly in her rocking chair in the next room. She found the music soothing. Sometimes she sat beside me on the piano bench. She said she loved watching my fingers move across the keyboard.

At the Smoky Hill school there had been a good deal of singing. In addition to being able to teach eight grade levels in one room, the teacher apparently was also required to play the piano. One of my favorite songs was "Billy Boy".

Oh, where have you been, Billy boy, Billy boy?

Oh where have you been, charming Billy?

I have been to see my wife.

She's the sweetheart of my life.

She's a young thing, and cannot leave her mother.

(Composer unknown)

(Pretty silly, those lyrics!)

But the student who sought me out in the wheat fields, nineteen-year-old Mozelle Clark, a senior at Bethany College, was offering me a whole new level of singing experience. For her senior thesis, she had determined to mount a production of Gian Carlo Menotti's Christmas opera, *Amahl and the Night Visitors*, originally commissioned by NBC for television. It would be the first college production of the popular opera in the nation.

She told me about her project and encouraged me to audition for the title role. Not until years later did Mozelle tell me how she had happened to come to me. She had asked around town if anyone could suggest someone to play Amahl. "Find Bobby Paulson," she was told. "He has the voice of an angel!"

Even had such a thought entered my mind, I would have been hesitant to try out. I knew that getting the role would mean I couldn't be on the team with my friends in the fall. But Mozelle was persuasive. She convinced me to audition and, ultimately, to take the part. "All the other boys can play football," she argued, "but only you can sing the role of Amahl."

It also helped that I immediately found the opera very appealing. The libretto tells the story of Amahl, a poor shepherd boy of about 12 who has a crippled leg and lives alone with his mother, who would be played by Mozelle. The Three Kings, who are following the Eastern Star to bring gifts to the Christ Child, come upon Amahl's hut and ask to spend the night. When Amahl learns of Jesus's birth and its meaning of peace and goodwill to all men, his crippled leg is miraculously healed. Stunned by this miracle, the kings invite Amahl to join them on their journey so Amahl can give his crutch to the baby Jesus as proof that he was healed because of his acceptance of Christ as his Savior.

Mozelle had given me a full copy of the music score for the audition when she came to the farm, and that evening I sat down at our piano to pick out the major singing roles. I discovered that the score contained duets between Amahl and his mother and trios among the Three Kings, all with quite beautiful harmonies. It would be enjoyable to sing, and it involved a lot of action and a lot of acting. Amahl was the central figure in the opera and remained onstage the whole time. You'd think the role might have seemed a bit intimidating, but I didn't see it that way, especially not with Mozelle's guidance and enthusiasm.

The story opens with Amahl's being mesmerized by the starlit night while his mother seeks to coax him to bed. After he settles in, there is a knock at the door. Impishly, Amahl tries to convince his mother that there are not one but three kings outside, "And one of them is black!" When she lets them in, Amahl's youthful curiosity leads to several exchanges with each of the kings, including a plaintive aria in which Amahl explains that he had been a shepherd but since his mother had had to sell all the sheep, they were forced to become beggars.

Although Menotti is Italian, he gave the music a decidedly

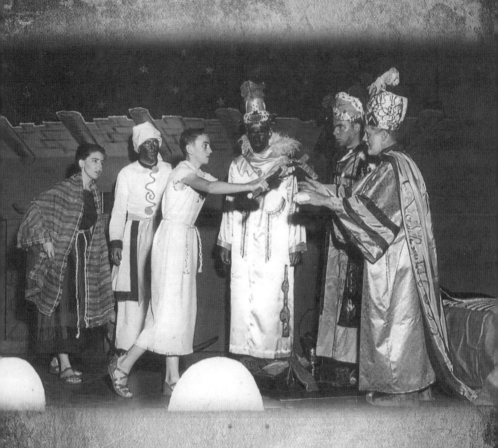

Scene from "Amahl and the
Night Visitors", Bethany College
production – from left Amahl's
mother (Mozelle Clark), Kings'
page (Louis Sherman), Amahl
(me, age 15) and the Three
Kings, Balthazar, Melchoir and
Casper (November 1952)

Middle Eastern feel by featuring the oboe in much of the orchestral accompaniment. The oboe becomes the voice of Amahl's wooden pipe, which he plays during the prelude while stargazing and in the closing scene.

I learned a good deal of the music before summer's end, much of it at my own piano. In addition, I met with Mozelle several times over the course of the summer at her parents' home in Lindsborg. She was my first voice coach/instructor. She taught me vocalizing exercises and we began to work on memorizing the pitches and pitch intervals in the Amahl role. During these sessions, Mozelle gingerly introduced me to the world of operatic singing: proper breathing techniques, voice placement and maintaining an open throat. It was a delicate balancing act. My natural singing voice was clear and bright, and Mozelle didn't want to change the freshness of the sound. Yet I needed to gain a measure of vocal strength and expansion of my vocal range to perform the role successfully.

As soon as college resumed in early September, the rehearsals began in earnest. At first, there were many rehearsals with piano accompaniment for just me and Mozelle. Later, we rehearsed the interactions between Amahl and the Three Kings, particularly King Caspar, who is slightly deaf and travels with a small box of treasures that greatly intrigues Amahl.

Then we began rehearsing almost daily to work out the staging, particularly the scene in which Amahl's mother attempts to steal some of the Kings' gold while they are sleeping in hopes of making a better life for Amahl. The Kings' page awakens just as the boy's mother reaches for the treasure, grabs her arm and shouts, "Thief! Thief!" Amahl comes to her rescue, fighting off the page and crying out, "Don't you dare! Don't you dare, ugly

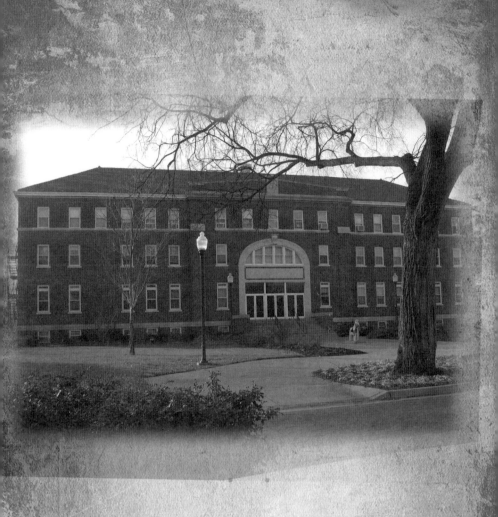

Presser Hall, Bethany College
campus (2008), and as it was
in 1952

man, hurt my mother!"

After individual scene and staging rehearsals, we had group rehearsals with the orchestra. All the while, Mozelle and all the college staff were terrified that my voice would change just before the scheduled performance in late November. As we worked out the timing, enunciation and correct pitch of the music, any time I spoke in a lower tone, everyone would jump.

"Is your voice changing?" someone might ask. Someone else might tease. "Don't do that again. You're making us crazy!"

In the meantime, Mozelle was busy writing press releases and sending them to numerous Kansas newspapers, printing up handbills, designing costumes and working with the art department to develop the scenery—even doing choreography for one scene in which a group of shepherds comes to Amahl's house to perform a dance to entertain the kings. Putting on this show was a very ambitious undertaking, especially for someone so young, just four years older than I.

Happily, my voice held up. The performance went off without a hitch before a packed house on the Bethany campus in Presser Hall, an auditorium with a large stage, space for a chorus of up to 400 and seating for nearly 2,000. For me at fifteen, the opportunity to mingle and work with dozens of college-age students and professors and to sing with an orchestra and conductor was an unusually maturing and life-changing experience. I have relished the memory of those few months all my life.

I remain in touch with Mozelle. Shortly after her graduation from Bethany, she married a classmate, Louis Sherman, who had played the role of the page in *Amahl and the Night Visitors*. She went on to obtain a doctorate in opera music and has enjoyed a fifty-year career in both religious and secular music production and performance.

Oh, yes: only a couple of months after the performance, in January 1953, my voice did change. Although no longer in the boy soprano range, I remained a lyric tenor for the rest of my singing days. (One of my school friends dubbed me *Tonsils* after my performance as Amahl, but thankfully the moniker didn't stick.)

I never played high school football again. The following year I took a part in a play put on by the junior class and, in my senior year, I traveled with the football team as an amateur sports reporter for the *Lindsborg News-Record*.

SOCIALIZING

Just like kids today, I spent my teen years *hanging out*.

Before I could drive, I socialized only on Friday and Saturday nights and only at the whim of Johnny or Arnold. They would give me a ride into town, and then I'd hang around the drug store or cafe until one or more of my friends showed up. Eventually, half a dozen kids might gather to roam the streets aimlessly.

Once in a while, we would go to the movies or sit in Pat's Cafe. Afterwards, my friends would go home and I would have to wait for my ride back to the farm, sometimes sitting on a curb or on the front steps of a store by myself for hours. It was not a perfect arrangement.

Sometimes we would go as a group to someone's house. Barbara Train's front porch was a popular meeting place. With her cute upturned nose and a friendly, outgoing personality. Barbara was popular with both the guys and gals. We also went to Karen Johnson's house. That was where I experienced the classic rite of passage for junior high school students—my first *spin-the-bottle* party.

Just as I was entering junior high, and timed perfectly for my enjoyment, Lindsborg had opened a Teen Town room on the second floor of an empty building a half block off Main Street. The large room held two ping-pong tables, a pool table, several couches, a jukebox and a dance floor. In that room, I learned to dance to Tommy Dorsey's "In the Mood," which was played dozens of times in the course of an evening.

On summer Wednesday nights during my high school years, I'd play my trombone in school band concerts at the band shell in the North Park. It was a good way to see my friends when school wasn't in session. Naturally, the Lindsborg swimming pool was a must for teenagers on summer Sunday afternoons. We swam, practiced diving and played water tag for hours. Mom often sat on the benches just outside the fence and watched. Those afternoons were a glorious experience, never to be repeated.

Once we were old enough to drive, we entertained ourselves with group trips to Salina for an evening of bowling or to McPherson for the drive-in theatre or the A&W root beer stand. It was tame but good fun, and we all enjoyed the camaraderie of our schoolmates.

TRAGEDY

In the small town of Lindsborg, our lives were generally carefree. So I was shocked at age fourteen to witness a tragic incident at the Lindsborg Pool a couple of years after it opened.

Shortly before the day it happened, I'd cut a fairly deep gash on the side of my leg. Since I was still bandaged up, I wasn't in the pool but sitting with my mother outside the pool fence. I still rue the fact. Had I been in the pool rather than a helpless bystander, there might have been a different outcome.

The Lindsborg Pool was a traditional rectangle, shallow at the end nearest to the entrance and changing rooms and deep at the other. The shallow portion extended to about two-thirds of its length, when it sloped gradually to a depth of five feet and then sharply to a depth of twelve. Several small, bullet-shaped buoys held aloft a rope that marked the transition from shallow to deep water.

Three diving boards—a one-meter board, a low board, and a three-meter board in the middle—were at the deep end.

On this late summer Sunday afternoon, the pool was packed. Suddenly, both lifeguards jumped down from their elevated chairs and ran to one side of the deep end. Within moments, they pulled out a limp body. Standing among the dozens gathered around to watch, I could see the lifeguards working furiously to pump out the water from the victim's lungs.

To my shock, I recognized him. He was a new friend of mine, sixteen-year-old Gene Lundquist. Gene came from a farming family that lived on the other side of Lindsborg from us, in a northwest area called Coronado Heights. His brother Donald, then about 18, was a powerhouse on the Vikings' high school football team.

When I was attempting to play football during my first year in high school, my locker was adjacent to Gene's, and we had had a few laughs together over the pre-school football practices. Gene was a funny, engaging kid who had enjoyed my self-deprecating humor regarding my football woes.

The lifeguards continued to pump for some 20 minutes. They didn't stop until Dr. Holwerda arrived at the pool, followed shortly by Gene's parents. Soon afterwards, Doctor Holwerda pronounced him dead.

It was an incredibly sad moment.

"Where were the lifeguards?" Gene's mother cried out. "Why didn't anyone see him? How could this happen? "

I could only clutch at the fence wire and shake my head in disbelief. There was nothing anyone could say, no sound but his mother's sobs as she crouched over his body. Then the ambulance came and Gene was gone.

Like everyone else in his family, Gene had been big-framed, tall and strongly built. He was well on his way to being the same kind of powerhouse football player as his brother. That's why his drowning was so perplexing. How could such a big and strong young person just drown *in plain sight*, so to speak?

We learned that Gene had been diving off the low board, doing mostly belly flops. Not a competent swimmer, he'd had some difficulty swimming to the ladder or the rope that marked the shallower water. During the autopsy, Dr. Holwerda found that Gene's lungs had been completely filled with the pool water. He surmised that Gene had attempted to take a big breath just before he entered the pool but instead took in water that might have caused him to black out. No one was watching to see if he surfaced after the dive, so he was floating on the bottom for several minutes before another swimmer spotted him and alerted the lifeguards.

When we dove with friends, we'd typically walk to the end of the board and check that whoever preceded us had swum away from the board before we made our own dive, especially if the person was an unsure swimmer. Our motivation was as much to protect ourselves as one another. If a diver lands on someone else in the water, both are hurt.

I regret that I'd been sidelined that day. Had I been with Gene, we probably would have been diving together. I believe I would have recognized his inexperience and would probably have noticed if he did not resurface after one of his dives. But that was not meant to be. I was not there, and Gene didn't get the help he needed.

EXTREMES

The pool was especially popular in Kansas because the summer weather was so hot.

For farmers, those hot, windy days in mid-to-late June and early July were crucial to ripen and dry the wheat kernels sufficiently to permit storing them and to dry the fields enough to allow harvesting equipment to operate. But they could make the summer days almost unbearable, even for a skinny kid like me. Frequently the temperature climbed well into the 90s, and it often reached 105°Fahrenheit and stayed there for as long as a week. "The hot wind just saps all my energy," Mom would say.

During nearly all of July and August, there was rarely a cloud in the sky. Sitting on the tractor, plowing, disking, and harrowing for most of those daylight hours, I would pray for any wisp of a cloud to pass over me and provide a moment's relief from the blazing sun.

Even at night, there was no respite. I vividly recall trying to sleep with the windows open wide, lying in a pool of sweat as I listened to the wail of the coyotes in the distance.

The winters were bad, too. Winters today are nothing like what I experienced in the mid-to-late 1940s and early 1950s. We suffered through temperatures as low as minus 26° Fahrenheit and accumulations of snow on our driveway at least three feet deep. When the county maintenance equipment plowed out the driveway, the piles of snow we'd play on afterwards could reach well over ten feet. And to get to town, we'd have to drive over frozen, windswept fields even to reach the main roads.

But extreme weather had its benefits for a child. We could enjoy ice-skating on the Smoky Hill River. It was great fun to fill our glasses with fresh snow, drop in a bit of vanilla extract, and have a vanilla shake. And only in the extreme weather did Mom allow us to bring our dogs inside!

But when you're a kid, you don't always think how treacherous the weather can be. My friend Herb Haskins and I were in high school when we decided to ice skate on the river from Lindsborg to Marquette. We hadn't gone far before my hands felt frozen. Herb began giving me his warm gloves while he took mine and attempted to warm them up between his hands, to no avail. We soon agreed this was a lame idea and turned back. Still, by the time we got back to my pickup, we had been out on the river for a couple of hours. My hands were so cold I could not turn on the ignition key. Herb had to do it.

I guess the temperature was about zero Fahrenheit. That

wasn't so bad, but overall, our plan—if it even deserves to be called that— was crazy dumb.

DRAFTED

The summer I turned 16 turned out to be a sad one for our diminished family.

Despite numerous appeals to the County draft board, Johnny, then 23, was officially drafted to serve in the Army in the Korean War. Mom was distraught beyond words.

"How could they? Don't they know I have only Bobby here to do all the farm work—milking the cows, feeding the pigs, plowing, harrowing, seeding, and harvesting the wheat? How will it all get done?" she fretted.

Arnold, a college student at the time, would be home during summer vacations to help with the plowing and to prepare for seeding. But since his acute asthma was particularly sensitive to the wheat dust, he had to minimize his exposure to the wheat harvesting operations.

I still remember the day Johnny got on line for the bus with a bunch of other draftees, all of them headed for basic training at Fort Leonard Wood, Missouri. Just like the others, he carried nothing but a small shaving kit. We all cried—Arnold, me, and especially Mom, who felt betrayed by the draft board and who best understood the gravity of our situation. Once again, she had the major burden of the farm to carry with only one part-time helper, twenty-year-old Arnold, and one full-time teenage worker—me.

WEATHER

Growing wheat on large acreages is like gambling with the weather. That's why on a farm, certainly in central Kansas, weather dominates all conversation and all farm activity and, to a great extent, determines how affluent a farmer will be. When I was growing up, it seems that some form of severe weather was always threatening.

Typically, the wheat harvest takes place in late June or early July. From then through most of September, time is spent plowing, disking, and harrowing the ground—smoothing the soil in preparation for seeding for the next crop.

Rain or hail in mid-June to mid-July can make the fields too wet for the machinery to harvest the wheat or create too much moisture in the wheat kernels to store them in grain elevators. If hailstorms occur after the wheat has matured and the seeds have formed, the hail can knock the heads of the individual wheat stalks to the ground, and the crop will be lost. Hail insurance cost nearly one-third of the value of a good crop, and every year, my mother would agonize about whether or not to buy it. She never did. Nor, I think, did our neighbors.

Winter wheat is planted in late September or early October. If there is sufficient rain, the young wheat will grow three or four inches and create a green velvet ground cover by late November or early December before the ground freezes for the winter. Then it should remain dormant until the spring.

If there is too much rain in the fall, the ground can't be prepared or seeded, but if rain is scant from October to November, the wheat won't have a good start before the freeze sets in. A good deal of snow is also desirable, as it helps get moisture into the ground during the spring thaw.

As the frozen soil begins to thaw, it becomes loose and crumbly. If ground cover has not been laid down, the loose soil will be picked up by the ever-present winds and create significant dust clouds. With John in Korea and Arnold at Kansas State, many times Mom would call me home from high school because one of the wheat fields was dusting. To keep the dust from *snowballing*, I would hook up the plow and actually plow one or two strips across the blowing dust, creating small moist ridges to hold dust that was loose. The technique was fairly effective.

Tornados were another cause for concern. Out in the field, we'd often see a dark cloud formation at a distance. If a small funnel began to extend downwardly, we quickly unhitched the plow or stopped working on whatever machine we were using and tore home as fast as possible. We'd duck into the underground cellar adjacent to the house and wait out the passing storm.

If rain, hail or tornados weren't on our minds, we'd be concerned about drought. It was a drought that precipitated the dust storms that caused such devastating economic problems in the thirties.

Though winds blow nearly constantly across the plains of the central states, prairie grasses hold the soil very well. But once the tractor replaced mules, ploughs with three or four plowshares in tandem replaced the single plow and ever-better machinery allowed the planting of more and more acres. As grasses were plowed under, greater swaths of bare soil were exposed in preparation for planting of crops—primarily wheat, the most lucrative.

The problem is that when soil becomes dry, there is nothing to hold it against the prairie winds. The extended drought in the 30s created the perfect conditions for a disaster but by the time

I was born, in 1937, the worst of the drought had passed. Our farm wasn't as badly affected as the western part of Kansas and the panhandles of Texas and Oklahoma, where large open fields had been plowed over. The crop fields around us were smaller, forty- or eighty-acre patches interspersed between patches of pasture and crops such as corn, cane, alfalfa, hay, and sweet clover. But the dust storms and lack of rain continued to be an annual spring concern.

Even without an actual drought, if rainfall was scant, the wheat wouldn't grow to its full potential and the crop would be slim, sometimes barely enough to provide seed for the next year's crop.

Despite all the potential hazards, I would guess that we had a really poor crop only about one year in five. We had bumper crops, when all the stars were perfectly aligned, about twice as often.

BUMPER CROP

One of our greatest crops was the result of a mistake.

In l953, as usual, the winter wheat crop was ripe and ready in early July, when the big combine crews that traveled from Texas to the Dakotas harvested it. Somehow, Arnold and I managed to get the plowing, disking and harrowing done before he went back to college at K-State. Then, it was up to me to seed the wheat for the next year's crop.

Wheat is planted using a drill with a series of discs spaced about three inches apart over a fourteen-foot length. A long triangular box extends across the length of the discs. The seed box has a series of holes in its bottom that are spaced in registry with the discs, and a long tube extends downwardly from each hole to a point immediately behind each disc. The discs are curved, like a wok pan, and the seeding tubes are located just behind the convex side of each disc. Finally, over each hole at the bottom of the seed box there is a metering wheel. As the drill is pulled along, it turns slowly, continuously feeding the wheat kernels through the tubes and into the small groove formed into the dirt by each disc.

When I'd finished seeding that fall, I put away the drill for the winter.

In early April or thereabouts, Mom decided we should plant a small crop of alfalfa, about 10 or 15 acres. She told me to use the same drill I'd used for the wheat. Shortly after I planted the alfalfa, we had several days of strong winds. All the local farmers began reseeding their alfalfa fields, worried that the initial seeding had blown away. I, however, did nothing because for some reason, my field didn't seem to be *dusting*—that is, the seeds weren't blowing away.

To compound the problems, the spring rains came too late. Our neighbors' alfalfa grew only spottily. Nothing at all was coming up in my field. Then, miraculously, my alfalfa appeared—in a full, luscious growth! The neighboring farmers were astounded.

In fact, I had made a fortuitous error. I hadn't known that winter wheat is planted with the drill disks set to make a furrow about three inches deep but that alfalfa seeds are planted at a depth of only about half an inch. When the late spring winds blew, the other farmers' alfalfa seeds blew away with the dust. Mine, on the other hand, were nestled comfortably under a couple more inches of dirt. When the spring rains finally arrived, my seeds were patiently waiting, and they sprang forth with gusto. Beautiful!

For years afterward, people talked about Bobby Paulson's amazing alfalfa crop.

TRANSITIONS

I was in high school when the era of rapid post-War growth began, thanks to a baby boom and a thriving economy. Though Lindsborg didn't experience the explosive suburbanization that transformed many areas of the United States in the late 40s and early 50s, our community had been changed in several ways by the time I left for college.

When I entered the Lindsborg schools in sixth grade, the whole school system was contained in a single city block. There were two two-story high brick buildings, one housing the grade school and the other housing the high school. Between them was a smaller building that contained a basketball court—a small one—and a stage. Through my junior year of high school, this is where we held junior high basketball games and school assemblies and where we put on orchestra and band concerts and our school plays. The buildings took up about half the block, and the remainder was used as a playground.

By my senior year, the new Lindsborg Rural High School was ready for occupancy, and its students included children from several small surrounding towns. It was built on the outskirts of the west side of town, about three blocks from the old high school, which then became a separate junior high.

The new high school—light-years superior to the old one— had a two-story, spacious gymnasium at one end and

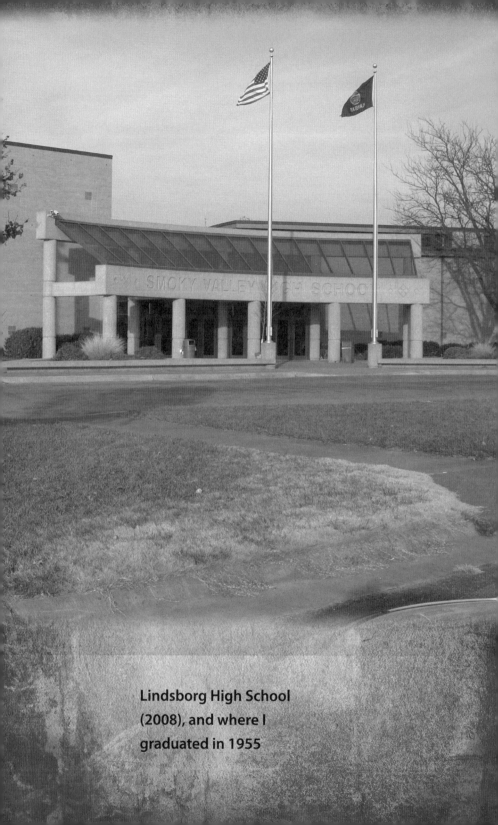

Lindsborg High School
(2008), and where I
graduated in 1955

an equally high and spacious auditorium at the other, with classrooms and administrative offices on a single floor in between. The auditorium had a large stage, room for an orchestra pit, and seating for perhaps two hundred people.

Within a year or so of the construction of the high school, Lindsborg had also opened a new, state-of-the-art community hospital, and the Bethany Church had built a two-story addition that housed classrooms for Sunday school, offices, and a large community meeting room.

Shortly after my high school graduation, Bethany College also began its transformation, which included building a new science hall and The Sandzen Memorial Art Gallery. Along with its permanent collection of outstanding works by Birger Sandzen, it shows the work of many local artists on a rotating basis. (Over the years, new classroom buildings and dormitories have been added, and today the campus covers a three-block-square area.)

The mid-to-late 1950s were halcyon days for Lindsborg.

OPPORTUNITIES

Though most of Lindsborg's robust growth occurred after I had left, it afforded me many opportunities remarkable in their depth and breadth for a town of only three thousand.

Performing in the college production of the *Amahl and the Night Visitors* opera was, of course, an eye-opening and confidence-building experience. But though there were only 33 students in my high school graduating class, we enjoyed no shortage of musical activities. I played a slide trombone in the school band, orchestra and brass ensembles, and I sang in choruses, quartets and octets. I also performed in our school plays, and though my football playing didn't amount to much, I was a member of the basketball and tennis teams.

I also had some first-rate instruction. Our English teacher, Einar Jaderborg, was working on his doctorate degree in English Literature from Columbia University. I have long been grateful that our math teacher, Gladwyn Dyck, encouraged us to check our calculations by roughly approximating the answers in our heads in order to rule out any answer that was clearly incorrect. Now there are plenty of handy mini-calculators, but I have continued to work numbers in my head all of my life. It's a good mental exercise.

We all benefited from the presence of Bethany College, which helped make Lindsborg a regional center not only for business, but for educational, religious and cultural affairs.

Along with basic chemistry, mathematics, and religion studies, the college offered high-quality music and art programs. Many area residents and farmers attended Bethany basketball and football games just to hear the Bethany pep band. The local churches supplemented their choirs with college student members, so the Sunday morning hymns were rousing, and the professor of organ music at the college, Lambert Dahlsten, a graduate of the Juilliard School of Music, was also the organist at the Bethany Church. Our Sunday morning services were richly enhanced by his beautiful renditions of intricate and thrilling sacred music etudes.

Bethany's professors Birger Sandzen and Charles Rogers, whose works are widely known, were just two of the several artists who called Lindsborg home. The administrators in the Lindsborg public school system *picked off* the best Bethany graduates to teach in Lindsborg.

The annual Easter Week productions of *Messiah* and *Passion According to St. Matthew*, with casts of hundreds, drew its participants and audience from all across the country.

But it wasn't just our hometown institutions that exposed me to a broad range of knowledge and activities as a youngster. My large family also taught me much. As a member of a working farm family, I learned how to use tools of every variety for repairing machinery, shingling a roof, building a fence, puttying a window, changing a tire and so on. Influenced by my sisters and brothers—Ruth playing the piano and John playing both the trombone and baritone—I, too, learned to play the piano and the trombone, read music and sing.

Though my mother struggled, I never felt deprived or envious of my peers. To the contrary, on the farm I learned to trust my own judgment, principles and abilities, and I vowed to become as self-sufficient and independent as possible. Somehow, I knew that if I could survive and compete on the farm, I could survive and compete in most anything. All that experience gave me the mettle I would eventually need to battle ALS.

As I look back on my early life on the farm and in the Lindsborg community, I marvel at the richness and diversity of my upbringing and look back to my childhood as a *Golden Age*. It gave me tremendous opportunities for self-improvement and developed my awareness of life's possibilities.

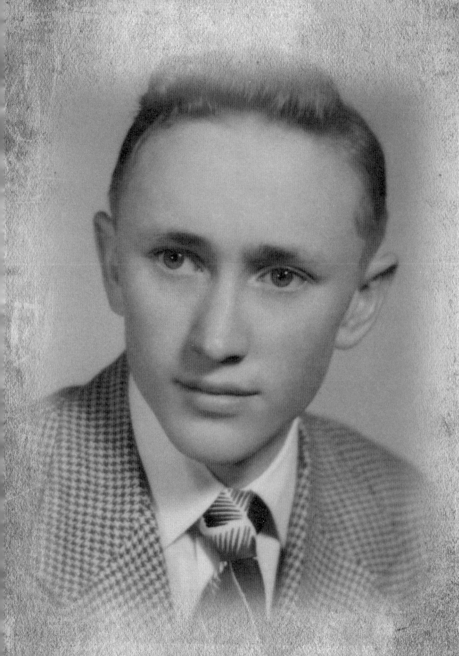

My brother Arnold, high
school graduation (1952)

K-STATE

My brother Arnold, the brains of the family, had gone to Arizona right after he graduated high school in 1952 to work as a carpenter's helper, building houses. The following year, having determined that rough carpentry work was not for him, he enrolled at K-State University in Manhattan, Kansas, about a two-and-a-half hour's drive from our home.

Our neighbor and former classmate in the one-room schoolhouse, Lloyd Ray Hanson, had run into Arnold one Saturday night. I recall Lloyd Ray as a typical young farmhand, and in my youth I had no inkling of his having had a religious calling, but he went on to become a Lutheran minister. A classmate of Johnny's went on to become a highly successful big-city surgeon. There were many stories of young farm boys and girls who went on to professional careers in many areas. And thanks to Arnold's serendipitous encounter with Lloyd Ray, my siblings and I would do the same.

Lloyd Ray, who was then probably in his last year of college or starting seminary school, had convinced Arnold that he could go to Kansas State for almost no money. At the time, Arnold had less than $200, no job, no books and no place to stay. (There were no men's dormitories until after we both had graduated.) And he'd wrecked his car, so he hitchhiked to Kansas State to enroll.

The salesman who gave him a ride to school advised him to study chemical engineering, and that's how he started out. But when K-State became only the second school in the country to be accredited for a curriculum in nuclear engineering, Arnold joined its first class of students to earn a Bachelor of Science degree in the field.

In mid-1955, Johnny came home from Korea, taking over the major responsibilities of the farm, so I was free to pursue other options. With a room to share and a job prospect for me, Arnold persuaded me to join him at Kansas State and to study nuclear engineering —cutting-edge technology at the time. At that point, he had been a student for two years, loved his college life, and knew all the ropes. I just had to follow along. "What's to worry?" was our attitude. I was ready to embark on my college career. I think I had forty dollars in my pocket!

But there was an immediate crisis. The job Arnold had lined up, waiting tables with him at an eatery in Aggieville — the neighborhood of bookstores, restaurants, beer joints and clothing shops adjacent to the university campus—fell through. The owner decided it wasn't smart to hire brothers, since we would be gone at the same time on holidays and school breaks. An emergency was averted when I got a job washing dishes at another restaurant two doors away. Like Arnold, I'd be working the dinner shift, from 5 p.m. until 7 p.m., and take my pay in meals.

So I was assured of having enough to eat, I could use most of Arnold's books, and a semester's tuition cost just $94, regardless of how many credit hours you took. That deal was especially helpful to me, since engineering students typically needed 18 credit hours per semester in order to graduate in four years.

Meanwhile, Johnny had been trying to make a go of the farm, supplementing his efforts with part-time work in nearby oil fields, but he was struggling. Swallowing enormous amounts of pride, he even went to Aunt Helga. She had the gall to let him rent only eighty of the 160 acres that she had wrongfully taken from our family.

Eventually, he decided to come to K-State also. When I started my junior year in the fall of 1957, he roomed with two other students and me.

Like Arnold—though with a bit more difficulty!—I managed to earn my own nuclear engineering degree, one of only seven students to do so in 1959. My fellow students, faculty advisers and professors at K-State were among the most intellectually gifted people I have ever known. I felt privileged to be in their midst.

PARTYING

I can't talk about Kansas State and Aggieville without mentioning the venerable and revered beer hall known as Kite's. As Morey's is to Yale, so was Kite's to K-State.

During four years of college and through four years of night law school later, my life consisted of study, study, study every waking moment, with few exceptions. The exceptions included Fridays at Kite's.

It was simply impossible not to stop in on Kite's on a Friday night in Aggieville—even for a serious student like me. Unfortunately for the science and engineering students, chemistry and other engineering laboratory classes were held on Wednesday and Friday from 2 until 5 p.m. The liberal arts students, who rarely had a Friday class past 3 p.m., could get a real head start.

We'd drink beer at Kite's, pitcher after pitcher of it, well into Saturday mornings. Since only 3.2% alcohol beer could be sold in a public establishment in Kansas at that time, it took twice as long to feel its effects! We spent most of Saturday sleeping off the Friday beer bash at Kite's. By 10 a.m. on Sunday, Arnold and I were at the local Lutheran church to practice with the choir, and an hour later, we were singing in our black robes.

On one occasion—and happily, only one—I overdid the boozing on a Saturday night. I was with a group of friends, one of whom actually lived in the college town. We were at his parents' home drinking beer and, intermittently, Scotch—not a good combination! But I got back to my room and made the Herculean effort to get to the church by 10 a.m. the next day despite my splitting headache.

As I was sitting with the choir in the front of the church, my stomach suddenly began churning. Right in the middle of the pastor's sermon, I had no choice but to get up, walk past the pulpit and down a side aisle, and then make a mad dash to the toilet in the basement. I got there in the nick of time. Everything in my stomach upchucked.

Phew. I had just barely avoided an incredibly embarrassing moment in front of the entire church congregation.

Did the good Lord save me? Had He decided I had done enough good deeds to be saved from such humiliation? Apparently so.

I had learned a good lesson. Scotch was not to be imbibed thoughtlessly and certainly not in combination with beer.

DEALINGS

During each of the summers following my first three years of college, I traveled to Denver, where I stayed with my sister Georgette and her husband, Oyer G., "Bill" Leary. Georgette worked for the Denver school system and Bill was a lawyer with the Conoco oil company. They lived in a Denver suburb, Thornton, of which Bill was also the mayor.

Bill's connections got me summer jobs working at the Conoco refinery near Denver, loading crude oil in railroad tank cars and gasoline in tanker trucks, and a part-time job as a lifeguard at the Thornton municipal swimming pool. My summers with Georgette and Bill allowed me to save nearly $1500 each summer, ample funds to see me through the school year in (almost) grand style! Without their help, my life story would have been quite different and far less full of adventure.

Through Bill, I also made one of the great investments of my lifetime. He took me to a used car lot somewhere on the seamy side of Denver, where I bought a 1941 Chevrolet for $40. All Bill wanted to know from the salesman was if the car had good brakes. However, when we brought the car home, my sister Georgette said, "Wait a minute. Did you remember to get a warranty?"

"For forty bucks, you expect the guy to give us a warranty?" He said exactly what I'd been thinking. We had a good laugh, and when Georgette realized how naive her question had been, she did, too. I drove the old '41 Chevy to and from the refinery that summer, back to Kansas in the fall, then back to Denver the next summer and I repeated the routine for one more year. At the end of the second summer, I sold the car to a junkyard for $25! That was one of the best investments I ever made.

In the meantime, Arnold earned spending money for college by continuing to work summers as a carpenter. Although it normally takes seven years to progress to the pay of a journeyman carpenter, Arnold reached that level by his third year of college. Each summer, as soon as exams were over, he studied a carpentry handbook and then jumped several levels in the carpentry tests.

Johnny, of course, received college money through the G.I. Bill, having served in the army in Korea. He also supplemented that income by selling Amana deep freezers with the company's novel home delivery food plan. If you purchased a certain monthly amount of meats and fresh vegetables for a year, the freezer was essentially free. But Johnny experienced a salesman's troubles. Though he would secure the housewives' purchase orders in the afternoon, by nighttime one in three might cancel when their husbands came home from work and calculated the amount of money that had been committed to the food plan.

DEBATE TEAM

A chance decision to join the debate team changed my life—though it almost cost me my life.

College registration in the 1950s was a hands-on affair. Each student sat with a counselor to work out a schedule of required and elective courses, and you had to make sure that the course you wanted hadn't been filled to capacity. Without computers, the procedure was laborious and maddeningly slow.

As the enrollment counselor went over my schedule, he suggested that I go over to the speech department. "Talk to Charlie Goetzinger about joining his debating squad."

I have no idea what prompted this remark, but I followed through. I found Professor Goetzinger to be an engaging and affable character and joined the team for the next two years. It was another valuable learning experience.

My fellow debaters and speech professors never failed to pick up a grammatical error, mispronunciation, or accent too colloquial to be tolerated. Until then, I had not realized that I had so many poor speech habits.

Debating competitions primarily centered on a topic of national interest and each team had to be prepared to argue either pro or con without advance notice. The competitions also included impromptu speeches, storytelling and poetry reading. When my professors learned I could sing, they put a guitar in my hands and I sang the ballad "Barb'ry Allen" at the next competition. It was a big hit. No other contestant had put poetry to music.

Since Kansas State was a land-grant college, participating in the Reserve Officers Training Corps (ROTC) was a mandatory requirement for two years. I was in the Air Force branch when I learned that the ROTC members on the debating team had been invited to a competition at the University of Pittsburgh's *high-rise campus*, a single multiple-story building named The Cathedral of Learning. I don't remember the outcome of the competition but the trip alone was an exciting adventure. My only other trip outside Kansas had been to Denver, and this was my first plane ride.

A debating trip to Dorado, Kansas was memorable in quite a different way. Five of us were packed into a car driven by one of our teachers, and I was sitting in the middle of the front seat. The roads were a bit slick from a recent snow. We hit an icy stretch and began to slide sideways. I sensed the driver was about to panic. I had experienced just such a situation many times myself driving the old pickup truck and knew there was only one thing to do. "You're okay," I said, trying to calm her.

"Just keep turning into the slide."

We slid right off the road into a fairly deep ditch, but the accumulation of snow cushioned our fall, and, as I had anticipated, no one was hurt. I knew that turning into the slide was better than turning away, which would have put the car into an uncontrollable spin and caused a potentially tragic outcome. Climbing out of the car and up to the road, my teacher and fellow passengers expressed their gratitude.

"Bob, we all were panicked, and then we heard your calm voice. You really saved the day!" I, too, was very pleased with myself.

TESTED

Though participating in the K-State debating team was fun, doing so while carrying 18 credit hours each semester in the nuclear engineering curriculum was academic suicide. My moment of truth came when I failed industrial stoichiometry, an absurdly difficult exercise in determining molecular weights of individual compounds or elements in a chemical composition. I bowed out of debating and repeated the course. Happily, I managed to get a B the second time, and industrial stoichiometry was forever behind me.

I have happier memories of chemical thermodynamics, which I took in the first semester of my senior year. There were fewer than a dozen students in my classes, and we all knew each other very well. Close to the final exam, a married student who probably had the best overall grade point average in the class invited several of us for a home-cooked meal followed by a final course review. Naturally, I accepted eagerly, as much for the food as for the study session. During the session, my fellow students helped clarify some of the points in my course work, so the evening was very productive.

As it happened, I received the highest grade on the final exam, assuring me an A for the course. When our papers were handed back and word of my achievement filtered out, I thought I detected some suspicious looks from my study mates.

"Hmm…," their expressions seemed to say. "How did he do it?" "Does he have an *in* with the prof?" I responded with only an innocent shrug of my shoulders.

FRAT BOY

Some of the most important lessons I learned at K-State were not in the classroom but in the fraternity house. But I valued the sillier times as well.

After I roomed with my brother Arnold for two years and with my brother John for a semester after Arnold graduated, I met Jim Lisher, "Lish". The pledge captain of Sigma Nu, he talked me into becoming a member. We roomed together for the rest of my college days and, since he too, pursued a career in New York, we have remained life-long best friends.

The Sigma Nu fraternity house where Lish and I lived at K-State has a stately perch atop a steep hill. Its front lawn slopes downward about 30 or 40 yards to the street. The house itself is a red-brick Colonial, and four two-story white columns frame the front door.

The three floors and basement of the house were all put to good use when I lived there. The basement was the hangout/party room, and the top floor was the primary sleeping quarters, filled with metal, military-style double bunk beds. The bunkroom windows were open in every kind of weather, making it the coolest room in the house in early fall and downright frigid in the winter months. Occasionally, we would wake up with snow on some of our blankets. But for just that reason, many of the guys preferred to sleep in the bunkroom rather than their individual rooms.

The second floor, dormitory-like, contained virtually all the student rooms, most with two beds, two desks and a closet. In the center of the floor was the single communal bathroom with eight wash-up sinks mounted back to back with a mirror above each, three or four urinals and the same number of commodes, and three or four showers. It was a busy place in the morning.

On the main floor, flanking the entrance hallway, were two rooms, one a living room perhaps 30 feet square and the other a dining room of similar size with six long dinner tables. Down the entrance hallway was a small suite of rooms that was the living quarters for the housemother, who was responsible for maintaining certain decorum—in the dining and living rooms, at least. The kitchen was located on the far side of the dining room, and on the far side of the living room were four more student rooms, usually reserved for the fraternity officers. A small room off the back of the living room contained a card table and a piano.

I felt privileged to be associated with the Sigma Nu fraternity but I had some hesitations as well. The house seemed pretentious and out of my league, and I often felt that being there meant that I was turning my back on my roots, on my mother, and on my farm life. So even though I lived in the house, I chose to be only minimally involved in fraternity affairs.

I was, however, at least superficially able to fit in. After all, nearly everyone was a Kansas hick, so how different or better than I could they have been? It helped that I had the right clothes. My sister Georgette and Bill loved to shop, so when I spent my summers with them in Denver, they saw to it that I had a suit, ties, sport jackets and slacks, all carefully color coordinated.

My brother Arnold never would have approved of my joining a fraternity—he was a confirmed "GDI", God Damn Independent, a status proudly claimed by many engineering students, who also proclaimed their identity by wearing a slide rule dangling conspicuously from one hip. I, on the other hand, carried mine on top of my stack of books. I didn't feel the need to call attention to what I was studying. (Since almost no one carried a backpack in those days, stowing it inside wasn't an option.)

At Sigma Nu, I learned from the housemother and upperclassmen the basics of proper table manners. Receive with the left hand, pass with the right (or vice versa). Bring the food to your mouth, not your mouth to the food. No elbows on the table. No hunching over your dinner plate. Cut with the fork in the left hand, knife in the right, then put down your knife and switch your fork to the right hand to eat. Wipe your mouth with a napkin before taking a drink of water between bites of food. Wait for everyone at the table to be served before eating. Don't leave a spoon in a coffee or teacup or a soup bowl, but replace it in the saucer. Don't talk with a mouthful of food. And chew with your mouth closed.

I also learned to shake hands with a firm grip, since nothing makes a worst first impression (on a man *or* a woman) than a limp handshake.

From our housemother, I learned how to treat a lady. Always open a door and let her go through first. Open and close car doors for the lady when she is getting into or out of the car. Walk on the outside, closest to the street, when you are accompanying her, and offer her your arm to hold. In a restaurant, allow her to order first. My debating partner, Kay Eplee added other tips—a lady shouldn't walk carrying a lit cigarette, and a man should always be ready to light her cigarette—but these are little used today!

The rules were observed in the living and dining rooms of the fraternity house, and both rooms were kept immaculate—by the pledges or *scerbs* as we called them at Sigma Nu. The rest of the house, particularly the second floor living quarters, was generally a shambles. In most rooms, clothes, books, shoes, papers, vinyl records, sports equipment, and other possessions were strewn around haphazardly. Lish had laid claim to an end room that was larger than most, and we shared it with a third roommate, Kent Salisbury. Since the three of us happened to be reasonably neat, I didn't have to endure the endless clutter in which the other fraternity brothers lived.

Hazing—that rite of passage from pledge to brotherhood in a fraternity—was fairly tame at Sigma Nu in my day. Serious injuries that had been inflicted during hazing in past years had forced college administrators to monitor it carefully and to threaten substantial penalties in the event of dangerous practices.

But the custom of *hazing week* had to be endured, not only by the pledges but also by the upperclassmen. On at least one or two nights, all the pledges were roused out of bed at about one o'clock in the morning and herded down to the basement where they were forced to partake in silly pranks, all designed for maximum harassment and embarrassment.

The pranks had names. Our fraternity chapter, Beta Kappa, specialized in one called "Bombardier." One pledge stood on a chair and cracked an egg on the head of a second pledge, then tried to drop the yolk into the mouth of a third pledge lying flat on the floor, face up. If the yolk just hit the face of the pledge on the floor, it counted for one point, and if the yolk hit the mouth, two. If the pledge on the floor swallowed the raw egg, three points were scored.

Another prank was the "Elephant Walk," which had some variations. First, all the pledges had to strip naked and then walk one behind another in a small circle. Then they were blindfolded, and told to walk "elephant style"—with the thumb of one hand in their own mouths and the thumb of the other between the "cheeks" of the fellow in front. That was bad enough, but then a brother would shout, "Switch!" which required the thumbs to be reversed. Ugh! The switching occurred numerous times for several minutes. Next, the pledges, still blindfolded, were told to pee while they continued to walk. One of the brothers then squirted warm water onto the backs of the legs of one or two pledges, evoking cries of "Oh, no, you bastard!" "Who did that?!" To the upperclassmen, it was great fun to see the trick successfully executed. The basement rocked with simultaneous howls of anguish and laughter.

Of course, cooperation in all the hazing antics was stimulated by lusty wielding of the paddleboards on the losing team or recalcitrant pledge.

Another favorite antic was to give each pledge a green food-coloring pill each day, turning the urine blue—a source of embarrassment when peeing in a public bathroom.

The most humiliating prank, however, required each pledge to carry a pencil and clipboard around the campus, and to approach women by saying "My pants were stolen. Do you have the hot pants?" and getting ten of them to sign. Of course, all the girls knew what was going on, and they usually cooperated with a generous smile. There was a hitch, however. The pledges were forced to wear an undergarment made from a scratchy burlap bag, and the pencil was tied to a string that passed down on the inside of the pledge's shirt and pants—and was tied to his penis. The string was just short enough so that getting each signature meant the poor guy had to endure several tugs on his privates, which were rubbing against the rough burlap. It took someone with a very fanciful imagination to concoct this particular indignation.

Aah, the fond memories.... I could go on, but these fraternity stories probably already are more than anyone wants to know.

However, there is a method to the madness of hazing. Forcing all the pledges to undergo the same humiliation built a bond that kept them close through their college years. (Who'd have guessed?) I still have my Sigma Nu paddleboard, Beta Kappa Brother 728, signed on one side by all of my pledge class and, on the other, by all the brothers in the fraternity.

Once we accept our limits, we go beyond them.

—Albert Einstein

Part Two: In the City

GROUNDWORK

By the end of summer, 1959, I had done the groundwork for my future life.

Since most of the students on the debating team were in a pre-law program, I had been inspired to cast my eye in that direction. Then, during my senior year of college, one of my engineering professors arranged for me to speak with his brother, an attorney who practiced patent law in Washington, D.C. Hooked by that conversation, I determined on a specialty in patent law. It would be a natural way to make use of both my engineering and law degrees.

One of my nuclear engineering professors put me in touch with the patent department of the Atomic Energy Commission (AEC) in Washington. I was offered a position, but there was a glitch. The job required "Q" security clearance that qualified me to see classified documents up to a top-secret level, and to process the clearance the FBI would need several months. (I later discovered that agents had conducted interviews regarding my general demeanor and activities with neighbors at our farm and even neighbors of my sister Georgette, with whom I'd spent my college summers.)

Mom co-signed a bank note so I could buy a used car

when I graduated, and in June 1959, I set out for the District of Columbia. Mom's advice was simple but sage. "When you get to Washington, just go and see our Senator, Frank Carlson. Maybe he can find something for you until you get your clearance from the AEC."

As soon as I arrived in Washington, I bought a newspaper and found a room in a three-story private home in the northwest section of the city, near the Sheraton hotel on Rock Creek Park—a very tony neighborhood, as it turned out. I used a map to orient myself to the District, and the next day I found the Senate Office Building on Capitol Hill. With the confidence of youth, I walked into Senator Carlson's office and approached the receptionist.

"Hi. My name is Robert Paulson, and I'm from Kansas."

"What can we do for you?"

"Uh, well, I'm here in Washington and looking for work for the summer. I have a job with the Atomic Energy Commission, but I have to wait two or three months for my security clearance. My mother said Senator Carlson might be able to help."

"He isn't in, but I can check with his legislative assistant. Wait here a minute."

A few minutes later, a young fellow emerged from a door behind the receptionist and introduced himself. "I understand you're looking for summer employment. Tell me more about why you're here."

I repeated my story, but he continued to look quizzical.

"What are you going to do for the AEC?"

"I'm going to work in the patent department and go to law school at night."

With that, the legislative assistant's face brightened.

"Perfect!" he exclaimed. "The Senator sits on the Post Office Committee. As you'll be a law student, he can justify your working in the legislative department of the Post Office. I'll get you the name and location where you should report."

Needless to say, I was ecstatic! Thanking the assistant profusely, I left in search of a phone to call Mom. She was very happy for me and especially pleased that our elected Senator had been so responsive to a constituent.

When I began working at the general counsel's office of the Post Office Department, the Senate and the Department were embroiled in arguments over some sticking points in a piece of legislation. I quickly became the designated messenger, picking up the latest draft from the Senate printing office in the bowels of the Capitol building and bringing it back to our general counsel—back and forth, back and forth.

I loved my little job. The secretaries, who were very accommodating, carefully explained that the cab ride to the Capitol would cost 25 cents and that I should tip ten cents but no more. Soon, I also became their proofreader. One of us would read while the other studied the copy with a hawk's eye. Every period, comma, semi-colon, capital letter and paragraph was read aloud. I was astonished at the speed, accuracy and dedication of those ladies.

Couriering the bills and postal replies back and forth, I learned the layout of the Capitol, Senate and House buildings, found the cafeteria frequented by the staffers and an occasional congressman, and familiarized myself with the train that ran beneath the whole complex.

Within a few months, I had graduated from college, bought a used car, driven to Washington, D.C., gotten a summer job and been accepted in the night division of the Georgetown Law School. By summer's end, I received my Q security clearance. All the pieces were in place.

LAW SCHOOL

In September 1959, I began working at AEC headquarters in Germantown, Maryland, about 20 miles northwest of the District, and I entered law school. A new, exciting era in my life had begun.

During the first few days of the semester at Georgetown Law School, which at the time was located in downtown Washington at Sixth and "E" Street, a student named Morris Yamner stood at the front door of the building. He had located a large, newly renovated and furnished apartment on "N" Street and was looking for roommates. He found Farrell Shaftel, Wayne Emery, and me.

I moved out of my day-to-day rental and into the apartment I'd share with my newfound friends. Morris, who grew up near New York in Passaic, New Jersey, was a graduate of Ohio State, and Wayne came from Pennsylvania and had gone to Harvard, but I can't recall the details of Farrell's background. Morris and Farrell were attending the day school, and Wayne and I were in the night division, so we'd graduate one year later.

I was very naive about life in the East and big city culture, but my roommates wasted no time initiating me.

I had found a Lutheran church during the summer, and on the first Sunday my roommates and I spent together, I invited them along.

"We're Jewish," Morris explained, indicating Farrell as

well as himself. "We don't go to church on Sunday."

I had never heard of such a thing. "When do you have church?"

"We go to synagogue on Saturdays," Morris replied.

I thought for a moment, then remembered, "But I didn't see you go anywhere yesterday."

"You're right," Morris explained, "That's a problem. Many Jewish people aren't very good at practicing their religion on a year-round basis."

We became a close-knit group. Wayne and I started class at 5:45 p.m. and were usually finished by 7:45, when Morris and Farrell often joined us for dinner. Morris was fond of scouting out new restaurants to try, and our meals were always jovial occasions with a lot of kidding and talk about our class work.

Law school was a delightful change for me. I had had so much math, geometry, physics and chemistry in college, all involving abstract formulas, equations, calculations, and chemical analysis, that I found it enjoyable to read instead about real people with real problems and practical, common-sense (most of the time!) solutions for governing their conduct towards each other in business and personal affairs.

In Washington, studying was a unique experience. On weekends, we could go to the main reading room at the Library of Congress or the sixth floor law library in the Jefferson Annex, just behind the Supreme Court building, probably the most architecturally beautiful building in Washington other than the Capitol itself. Sitting among these hallowed buildings, with the whole history of our country literally at my fingertips, was inspirational.

I had still another option for quiet study. Although my desk was outside the District at headquarters, a sprawling complex with four separate wings, the AEC also had a set of executive offices (including a small law library) in downtown Washington. On weekends, the downtown offices were deserted, so I had the law library all to myself.

To keep up with the class work, I had to study for two hours each night after dinner, plus at least 10 or 15 hours over the weekend. The crucial time was about 9 or 9:30 at night. The temptation to just lay back and relax on the bed for a moment was strong, but if I succumbed, the next thing I would hear would be my alarm at 7 a.m. So, each night after dinner, it was imperative that I go straight to my desk. It sounds onerous now, but everybody I knew was doing the same thing at the time, so it seemed normal.

In my early thirties, I worked with a young lawyer in California about my age, who had attended Harvard Law School. He said that he'd gotten through Harvard by studying every waking minute of every day with the exception of the two hours he spent having dinner with his wife on Saturday night. I realized I wasn't the only one who'd felt obliged to study non-stop in law school.

TASTES

In his ongoing quest for a good restaurant, our roommate Morris expanded our gastronomical horizons.

The Black Angus Steakhouse was always a favorite, even though it conjured up memories of my own less than successful adventures with Blackie the calf! The steaks were aged and well marinated, and the baked potatoes came with extras that were something of a novelty in those days—sour cream, chives, and crumbled bacon bits. During my law school years, from 1959 to 1963, the whole meal probably cost less than eight dollars.

A more modest establishment, the coffee shop in the Mayflower Hotel, was a place I will never forget. There was table seating but we preferred to perch at the counter. Manning the grill was a large, jovial woman, probably in her mid-forties.

We loved to watch her work on her masterpiece: the club sandwich. She'd place the bacon strips on the grill, then pop the bread into the toaster. When the toasted bread emerged, she'd slather it with mayonnaise, add fresh slices of tomatoes and baked chicken strips, and top it all off with the freshly grilled bacon. Our mouths would water as we watched. Was it the freshness of the ingredients that made it so delicious? All I know is that I have never had that club sandwich's equal.

Some years later, I returned to the Mayflower, hoping to recapture the experience I so fondly remembered. To my great disappointment, both the grill lady and counter were gone, and an upscale restaurant had replaced the coffee shop. Sometimes, a change doesn't represent progress.

Can there ever be too much of a good thing? The answer is yes, or so I learned at the Sheraton Hotel, adjacent to the Rock Creek Park in Washington. Morris had discovered that the hotel set out an unbelievable smorgasbord of food for Sunday brunch at the all-inclusive price of four dollars! The round appetizer table alone had four or five tiers. There was also every type of fish, beef, pork and chicken entree imaginable, plus desserts, all set out on separate tables.

We did what you might expect of a group of 22- and 23-year-olds. We tried not to eat on Saturday and then went to the Sheraton on Sunday to gorge ourselves. Such erratic consumption took its toll. The following day, we all suffered from stomach aches.

On my payday, we went very upscale and made dinner reservations at Francoise's, a French *snob eatery* a couple of blocks from the White House across Lafayette Park. It may have been pretentious, but I loved it. It was where I first tried snails—*escargots*—and I was immediately hooked on the garlic-and-butter sauce, garnished with a touch of parsley, in which they were cooked. It was a far cry from the hamburgers and ketchup at Pat's Cafe in Lindsborg.

NEW YORK

My roommate Morris not only introduced me to fine dining, he also gave me my first taste of New York City.

During the summer break after my second year in law school, he invited me to come to Passaic one weekend and stay over at his parents' house. Early on Saturday evening, accompanied by two of Morris's friends from New Jersey, we headed for Manhattan.

As we made the last long turn from New Jersey's Route 3 into the Lincoln Tunnel, Morris made sure I looked over the Hudson River to the New York skyline. It was—and is—a stunning view, especially to someone who grew up on the flat plains of Kansas.

Morris and his friends gave me the complete city tour, including stops at the Brooklyn Bridge, the Empire State building, Central Park, the Waldorf-Astoria Hotel, Times Square and Greenwich Village.

Having spent summers in Denver and lived in Washington for a year, I had had some experience with good-sized cities. However, nothing prepared me for the awesome height of the Empire State building. Morris and his friends laughed as I stared, mesmerized, at the giant structure. "See," they all said at once, "We told you! You can't help but stare the first time! Nobody can!" Years before, I had read a news report of a military plane flying into the 77th floor and had been astonished that the building didn't topple over. Now I could see why it didn't. When I looked at the building up close, I realized that the light plane would be no match for the tremendous bulk of steel, concrete and stone contained in the broad base of its walls.

Driving through Times Square and the theatre district, I was struck by the mass of people thronging the whole area. I had never seen so many people at one time. It was intimidating but also exhilarating. I couldn't wait to be part of the whole scene.

Strolling on Greenwich Street in the Village, I was greeted by yet another unfamiliar sight—men holding hands. Then I learned that the Village was a haven for homosexuals, but that no one really cared. I liked New Yorkers' attitude: *Live and let live.* It was, and is, as simple as that.

At the end of the evening, well past midnight, Morris and his cohorts decided I should see Harlem. Soon, we were in a bar in the very center, on the corner of 125th Street and Lenox Avenue. This was 1961, nearly fifty years ago, and four years before Martin Luther King's march in Selma, Alabama. Even today, race relations are not always as cordial as they should be, but back then, things were extremely dicey. We didn't have any business in that environment.

We had been in the bar for only a few minutes before half a dozen or more prostitutes pressed their faces up against the windows, motioning us outside. Several police walked by, chasing the women away, but once the cops were gone, back they came.

Morris and his buddies were a gregarious group, and they easily struck up a conversation with several black men on the way back to our car. Their mentioning that I was from Kansas evoked some broad smiles. Coincidentally, "Kansas City" was a popular song at the time. "Hey, Kansas," they called to me, "You're a long way from home, but you must be a good guy. We love Kansas City!" I didn't bother to explain that my hometown was far from there; I was just happy to be accepted as a Kansan.

Just as we were getting back into our car, a pair of cops came by. One came over to Morris and softly admonished us. "You fellows need to get out of here. This is no place for you."

Driving back to Washington the following day, I heard the familiar song lyric running through my head: "New York, it's a helluva town."

Throughout my first years in New York, I remained in close contact with Morris. He continued to offer tips on city living, often met me for dinner on the weekend (at restaurants he chose), and introduced me to shopping at wholesale prices on the Lower East Side (mainly Orchard Street just off Delancey) and in the garment and jewelry districts.

Along with my future roommate Hal, Morris gets credit for helping to school me in how to make one's way in the Big Apple.

LAUNCHED

Four years of night law school seemed daunting at the beginning, but—as with all of life—the years passed all too quickly.

As if the challenge of school itself wasn't enough, I heaped on more. I was apparently a glutton for punishment. Though I should have learned from my debating experience in college that extracurricular obligations can be disastrous, when my grades in law school were good enough to qualify for the Georgetown Law Journal, I accepted. But this decision was a good one.

The entire legal system in America is built on following precedent known as *stare decisis*. Consequently, a rigid, excruciatingly detailed set of rules has developed for citing prior case law decisions, legal treatises, statutes, Congressional comments, and so on that are argued to support a legal proposition or position. These rules are set out in a small, thick handbook known as the *Blue Book of Citations.*

As a staff member of the law journal, I was obliged to review articles submitted for publication by professors, judges or legal practitioners, to read every piece of precedent referred to in the article, to confirm that it indeed supported the author's proposition, and then to be certain the precedent was properly cited. This procedure often required the efforts of other staff members and, sometimes, heated discussion to resolve the issues. The work was invaluable training in writing a legal brief that was clear, concise, and persuasive.

When you're working so hard, you really enjoy any sort of comic relief. That's probably why I recall so vividly a fellow student's tale of a Halloween gone wrong. Instead of buying candy, he'd decided to hand out oranges to trick-or-treaters as a healthy alternative. When a little four-year-old girl showed up among a group of costumed kids and held open her bag, my friend proudly dropped in an orange. The little girl looked into the bag, and then looked up accusingly. In her tiny voice, she angrily said, "You son-of-a-bitch, you broke my gingerbread man!"

I also remember when a student who knew a little bit about golf insisted that three of us who were total novices join him. Needless to say, the afternoon was largely spent searching for lost balls. We were teeing off from the men's position, some 10 or 20 yards behind the ladies', which was marked by a small, square wooden block on either side of the space. Our friend was already exasperated. With all his might, he blasted the ball off the tee. It went straight along the ground, struck one of the small blocks and bounced back over our heads, landing behind a split-rail fence. It must have been the only time a golfer produced a lost stroke, negative yardage and an unplayable lie on his tee shot!

Graduation in June 1963 was mighty sweet. The day was clear and warm, Mom flew to Washington for the ceremony, and Arnold drove up from Virginia. It was a proud day for all of us. I was especially pleased that my mother, then 70, had made the trip.

Only two months or so before graduation, I had happened upon a hallway conversation among several classmates discussing job opportunities. One, Ed Fitzpatrick, had transferred to New York's Fordham University Law School the year before, and he began telling the group about the patent law firms he knew of in New York. In particular, he mentioned that the young firm Morgan, Finnegan, Durham and Pine was hiring new law graduates. I arranged an interview and was hired.

I started work with the firm in July and remained there almost 40 years, until ALS forced my retirement in June 2003.

THE BAD OLD DAYS

I arrived in New York on July 4, 1963 and began work at Morgan Finnegan four days later. At the YMCA on the corner of Ninth Avenue and 34th Street, just a couple of blocks from Macy's, I took a room with a bath—a wise decision.

All of my worldly possessions were in the car I had bought just before I left Washington, a new 1963 Chevrolet Impala convertible. That, as I would learn, was an unwise decision. As I parked my car in a lot next door, I off-handedly asked the attendant if my stuff would be safe. Eyeing my suit jackets hanging in the back seat, he hesitated. "Well—what size are you?"

Ever the innocent, I replied, "38 Long."

"Don't worry, then," he said. "You're not my size."

Less than reassured, I left the car anyway, and suffered no loss that night. I would not be so lucky over the next two years.

I'll try to give a snapshot of New York City when I arrived in 1963. Fifth and Madison Avenues were two-way streets. There was no Tavern on the Green and there were few outdoor cafes and restaurants. Max's Kansas City was the "in" restaurant, and discotheques were the hot new thing— especially Shepherds in the Drake Hotel at Park Avenue and 52nd Street. There was no Dumbo, SoHo or Tribeca. An eight-room coop at the Dakota sold for $30,000 (though the monthly maintenance fee of $790 was steep), and a studio apartment in a doorman building midtown rented for $165, but you could get a place in the East

Village for $45 a month. You could take out a dollar bill, pay for an egg salad sandwich and a Coke at the five-and-ten-cent store lunch counter, and get enough change to leave a tip and put some back in your pocket. The ideal date was an airline stewardess, because you could be sure she would be young, vivacious and knowledgeable in the "ways of the world."

But the quality of life was not so great in many ways. The subway cars weren't air-conditioned, and there was no way for anyone in a wheelchair to get on a bus. Every building burned trash in incinerators, so the air was full of tiny round balls of soot that would collect on windowsills every day. Coming back to the office after lunch and a short walk, we checked our faces in the bathroom mirror for soot on our noses, and I squinted to keep the flecks of soot and paper bits floating in the air out of my eyes and away from my contact lenses.

Crime in New York at that time was rising, and it would escalate through the 1970s and into the 1980s. The top of my convertible was slashed twice. Finally, I simply left it unlocked, another bad idea. I bought a new set of tires and the next morning they were replaced with four bald ones. (The thieves were remarkably thoughtful). The unlocked car was stolen and recovered twice, then stolen a third time for good. When I asked if the detective had any information, he said, "Believe me, Mr. Paulson, if we locate the car, you'll be one of the first to know!"

Break-ins were common. So were robberies and muggings. "Squeegee men" gathered at stoplights to wash a car windshield while the driver waited at a red light. If a woman driver rolled down her window to give a tip, the window-washer might rip the necklace off her neck or grab her purse.

The situation reached some kind of peak in 1984 with the

attempted mugging of Bernie Goetz, an electronics specialist riding the subway to work just like two or three million other New Yorkers. Goetz, who had been mugged before, was carrying a gun. When four teenagers approached him with sharpened screwdrivers, he didn't hesitate to use it, crippling one of his attackers permanently and wounding the others, some seriously. All the victims had prior criminal convictions. Eventually, Goetz was convicted of a misdemeanor for carrying a concealed weapon, and he served nine months in prison.

Known as the *subway vigilante* incident, the Goetz affair vividly demonstrated how lawless the city had become, and there was a public demand for action. The second half of my 45 years here in New York has been far more pleasant than the first. Subways are safe, air-conditioned and relatively clean, no incinerators pollute the air, indigents aren't harassing drivers, and the incidence of vandalism, car theft, and muggings is down. For this old-timer, nowadays is a definite improvement over *the old days*.

LODGING

New York may have had its share of undesirable elements in the 60s and 70s, but it was an exciting, vibrant and fun place to live and work, and I didn't want to be anywhere else.

Once again, I got lucky.

I had decided it was time to leave the Y. Though I knew I couldn't afford an apartment on my own, that didn't appear to be a problem, since it was customary at the time to have a roommate or two. At Georgetown, people had posted notes on the law school bulletin board to announce that they were looking for apartment shares. I decided to check out the New York University Law School bulletin board to see if that were the case here.

Sure enough, I found a notice. When I called to ask about the apartment, the fellow who answered asked how I'd gotten his number.

"Off the bulletin board," I explained.

There was pause at the other end. "I should have taken that note down, because I did have a guy staying with me," said the voice, "but he changed his plans. So—why don't you come by tomorrow night?"

And that's how I met Harold—known as Hal— Zinn.

His place was at 45 West 10th Street, at the northern end of Greenwich Village. Though officially it was a one-bedroom apartment, Hal had walled off most of the living room area to make a second bedroom, leaving a tiny area for a living room and entrance with a couch. The rent was $415 a month, but Hal asked me to pay $215, since he had provided the furniture. I readily agreed.

In the 60s, the city was undergoing a tremendous spurt in construction, and Greenwich Village had its share of new apartment houses. It also had a large stock of relatively inexpensive housing, much of it in ramshackle buildings that dated to the turn of the century and before. So there was a particularly rich stew of people from every walk of life: Rich and established gentry on lower Fifth Avenue and in townhouses facing the park at Washington Square. Working-class families of Italian immigrants who'd settled the neighborhood several decades before. A polyglot mixture of students and professors attracted to New York University from all parts of the world.

Gays, lesbians, and cross-dressers feeling welcomed in the freewheeling atmosphere of the intimate streets. Famous jazz, rock, and folk musicians who performed on Bleecker Street at nightspots like The Bitter End and The Village Gate. Actors plying their craft at a burgeoning group of off-Broadway theatres. And artists taking advantage of large, cheap studio spaces.

The locals who lived there and the out-of-towners who came to gawk mingled at a wonderful variety of ethnic restaurants, small cafes, coffee houses, and bars. Hal introduced me to several: Peter's Backyard, directly across the street from our apartment, known for its steak dinner. The Ninth Circle, where the shells of peanuts served at the bar littered the floor. Minetta's Tavern, for its authentic Italian food and The Elephant and Castle for its hamburgers. The bar at 17 Barrow Street, now One If By Land, Two If By Sea, one of New York's most romantic dining spots. The legendary speakeasy Chumley's, demarked only by a single yellow light bulb over the door.

I once read that a newcomer in small towns takes years to be accepted in the community, if indeed it ever happens, but that in New York, after a few return visits to the neighborhood restaurant, diner, cleaners or drug store, a new arrival is quickly accepted and greeted as an old acquaintance. I can vouch for the truth of that statement.

Hal and I shared the apartment for nearly two years while he completed law school and a summer internship with the U.S. District Attorney's office. He turned out to be a great roommate for me. He had grown up in a nearby suburb on Long Island and had a large network of friends as well as three younger brothers. I was very busy at work, and at home there was a constant stream of Hal's friends and brothers coming and going, so I never had to worry about being lonely.

Tall and athletic, a *scratch golfer* who played the course at par, good-looking enough to attract girls easily, Hal was single-minded in his quest to find *the right one*. On the street, in a restaurant or a bar—and even through a taxi window!—Hal managed to get girls' phone numbers. There were no computer dating services or *speed dating* events in those days, but Hal had his own system. For first dates, he'd only take the girl to lunch, thus ensuring he wouldn't *waste* more than two hours if the conversation wasn't stimulating. Before the lunch was over, Hal always managed to grill his date thoroughly, extracting all the details he needed about her family background, education, religion, goals, line of work, interests, and so on. I hadn't met anyone like him before; nor have I since.

Once Hal completed his law clerk internship, he moved to London to pursue employment recruitment, sensing that a computer-based system would be a powerful asset and knowing it wasn't yet in place in England. (I think he should have started a computerized dating service, considering his expertise in the area.)

His leaving New York meant I had to find another place to live.

CONVERTIBLE

One of the ways you could tell I wasn't a native New Yorker was that when I arrived, I kept a car in the city.

The parking problem alone discouraged car ownership. For three years—before my Chevy convertible was stolen for the last time—I had to deal with New York's alternate-side-of-the-street regulations. New at that time, they were and continue to be a pain, but much of the time I managed to sidestep the hassle of moving the car from place to place by driving to work. My offices were downtown at 80 Pine Street, on the corner of Water Street, close to Wall Street and to the East River. The area has since been built up, but at the time, the only local landmarks were the Fulton Street Fish Market, a seafood restaurant known fondly to its patrons as *Dirty Louie's*, and a lot of parking lots. I found one on Water Street under the Brooklyn Bridge that charged just $1.50 a day. Still, that was a bit of an extravagance, since a subway token then cost just 15 cents.

In addition to the parking issues, the incidence of car theft and vandalism in the early 60s also made car ownership problematic. Certainly no local would be foolish enough to buy a convertible because it was such an easy target. But I fondly recall how the fact I owned one—black, with a red interior— made it easy to impress the stewardess I was taking on a tennis date one sunny summer Saturday. I had a tennis permit—a season's permit cost $15—and we were driving uptown with our racquets in the back seat.

"I can't believe I'm riding in a convertible with the top down in New York, driving up Fifth Avenue to play tennis in Central Park," she exclaimed, throwing up her arms as if to embrace the whole world as her very own. Later, we danced the night away at Shepherd's, my favorite discotheque.

Having a convertible also attracted other, unwelcome attention. On another warm Saturday night, I was driving up Third Avenue alone with the top down. Stopped at a red light, I suddenly found myself next to a group of four women, obviously *ladies of the night* looking for a cab.

"Hey, handsome," said one of them, leaning against the car door. "How about a ride uptown for us girls?"

"Sure, why not?" I heard myself say. "Hop in!"

They tumbled into the car, chattering excitedly, two in the back seat and two beside me. (There were no bucket seats in those days.)

"Now, this is living!" I heard from the back seat as we rode along.

"Gee, you're a sweet guy," said the girl next to me. "We're going to a party on 96th Street. Why don't you come along?

I declined graciously, having decided that this episode might go very wrong. I took them to their party and breathed a sigh of relief when they all piled out.

Throughout my years in Washington and for the first couple of years in New York, I kept Kansas plates on my car. That was tantamount to having diplomatic immunity. Without computers to track down parking violations, tickets on an out-of-state license plate could be largely ignored. Still, there were limits on how far I would go. In Brooklyn, I definitely did not park when the sign read "DO NOT EVEN THINK ABOUT PARKING HERE." Now *that* was a traffic sign that clearly made its point.

My Kansas plates saved me big-time one lunch hour at about 48th Street and Madison Avenue, which was then still a two-way street. Rushing to pick up a pair of trousers that had been altered, I double-parked, ran into the store, returned to the car and then made a U-turn to save time getting back to the office. When I got to the first intersection, a cop directing traffic motioned me to pull over.

"You think I didn't see you double park and then make the

U-turn? Gimme your license!"

I handed it over. He obviously noticed it was from Kansas, and then he checked my plates.

"What are you doing here?"

"I work here," I said meekly. "I'm on my lunch hour."

The cop sighed, exasperated. "You've broken so many laws, I'd spend a day writing you up. Just get the hell outta here—and don't do that again!"

MAUREEN

Luckily for me, I wasn't at loose ends in my convertible for very long.

Since we had become roommates, I was often the beneficiary of Hal's relentless quest to find the right girl. "Bob," he'd say, "I had lunch today with this very cute girl. She's not for me, but I think you might like her. Give her a call."

And his connections led me, eventually, to Maureen. The first girl I met through Hal was named Pat, and through her, I met Betty Leonardo. Betty had one group of Irish friends who went to the Jersey shore and another—acquaintances of Maureen's, I later learned—who shared a summer rental house in the Hamptons.

Betty and I dated casually over the course of two summers, during which time she occasionally mentioned yet another group of girls with whom she had traveled to Cape Cod and gone skiing in Vermont and Colorado. During the late summer of 1968, she said two of them were having a dinner party at their apartment on East 83rd Street. She invited me to come along and bring another guy, so I brought my Kansas frat buddy, Jim Lisher.

Maureen was one of the girls hosting the get-together, a large, friendly group of perhaps ten or twelve. Although there were an even number of men and women, no two of them seemed to be paired off, and conversation was free-flowing and spirited. Though Jim and I were newcomers, the girls all seemed to enjoy our company. I had stepped into a world in which I immediately felt comfortable.

Within a few days of the dinner party, I met Maureen and her roommate Mary Lou for a hamburger at Martel's on Third Avenue and 83rd Street, then a *hopping bar*—one of the places where the younger set of Upper East Siders dropped in regularly. We seemed to have a lot to talk about—certainly I did; I probably told my farm stories—and I was happy when Maureen asked me to accompany her to a friend's wedding the following weekend.

The wedding date didn't have the best ending. The hosts plied me with far too many drinks and Maureen had to drive us back to the city after I bounced off a curb on the way to the parkway. The rest of the evening is a blur. Nevertheless, Maureen accepted a subsequent date with me. I took her to L'Orangerie, a popular restaurant of the period, and I brought her back to see my apartment before walking her home. From then to the end of 1968, Maureen and I were together at every free moment, dining out, partying with her friends, cooking dinners at my place for her roommates and their dates, and even visiting with her parents and her parents' friends.

"This is a very classy broad!" I thought. I liked her looks and I liked her figure: tall, shapely, and yet strongly built. I liked her hairstyle: short on the neck, long in front with a flip over one eye. I liked the way she dressed: tailored, with no frills but with lots of flair. She often wore slacks and a blouse, sort of a Kate Hepburn look, plus open-strapped, high-heeled shoes that accentuated her ankles. I recall a snappy belt here, a little pin there, and, on her right wrist, a smart, wide, brushed-gold bangle bracelet (a gift from a former boyfriend, I would later learn).

For Christmas 1968, Maureen invited me to spend the holiday with her parents at her uncle's house in St. Petersburg, Florida. It was a romantic, fun-filled few days, and it was there that I proposed to Maureen over wine at the Thunderbird Hotel lounge on the beach. She accepted, and I was subsequently glad I'd done the asking then, because two days later, I made a bit of a fool of myself in front of her.

We had driven across the state to visit friends who owned an oceanfront motel in Vero Beach. Years ago, in the Lindsborg pool, I had perfected a trick dive, pretending to fall off to one side of the board on the second bounce. When I tried the same trick at the motel pool, my left foot caught the board, severely twisting my ankle. I tried to shrug it off, but within an hour my ankle had swelled up noticeably, and I was in excruciating pain.

By early evening, Maureen's dad determined to check me out with an X-ray. Although it showed no break, I was in such agony the emergency room nurse said she would give me a "double whammy" to take the pain away—not pills, but an injection. Just as I reached the car in the wheelchair, I threw up and then blacked out. Maureen and her dad carried me into bed in our room and I didn't wake up until the next afternoon! My embarrassment was nearly as bad as the pain, but I thought that if Maureen and her parents could handle me at my worst, I guess we were meant to be together.

HOME

Instead of remaining in the Village after Hal's departure, I decided to move to the Upper East Side. There I found the place that would truly become home.

After the Third Avenue El was torn down in the 1950s, lots of new buildings had gone up in the Upper East Side from about 59th to 86th Streets. Many of them were white brick buildings with a large number of studio and one-bedroom apartments. These offered, for the first time, a large stock of housing suitable for young, single people who—up until World War II—tended to live with their families until they were married.

So the Upper East Side had a large population of young, single people. Crowds of them hung out in a long stretch of bars along Second Avenue, especially at the then-new TGIF's and Maxwell's Plum. On Third Avenue, Malachi's was so packed, there was no place to sit, and a trip to the bar and back to a spot to stand took up most of the evening.

For several weekends, I looked for my own apartment in the neighborhood, hoofing back and forth between Lexington Avenue and First Avenue on the side streets in the entire two-mile stretch, asking doormen or superintendents at each building if anything was available. Somewhere along the way, I realized I should be looking at buildings close to a subway express stop so I could get downtown to work as quickly as possible. The apartments near the 59th Street stop were too expensive, so I decided to look in the area around 86th Street.

I was fortunate to find an apartment on 86th Street between York and East End—and 43 years later, I'm still there. It's in the heart of Yorkville, an area that once was heavily populated by German immigrants and where Lou Gehrig, whose parents were

German immigrants, grew up. When I moved in, there were several German restaurants remaining along 86th Street as well as the popular Lorelei German dance hall. The Turn Verein, an old German community center, remained on Lexington Avenue and 85th Street until 1985.

The apartment I found was perfect for me. A so-called junior one-bedroom, it had a large living-room area with a wide expanse of windows overlooking the park, the East River and the Triborough Bridge; a separate small bedroom; a large bathroom (perhaps eight feet square); and a small galley-style kitchen.

I bought a standard double bed mattress on rollers, and one of my associates at the firm gave me an old headboard in exchange for a game of tennis on a private tennis court near his house in Oyster Bay, Long Island. Morris's grandmother had recently died and he gave me her outdated living room furniture: a dark green velvet couch (Victorian style, tufted back with curved armrests), a large velvet wingback chair, a couple of end tables, and table lamps. I bought a flimsy round table and six flimsy ladder-back chairs at The Door Store for a dining-room area at the end of the living room opposite the windows. I had fully furnished the apartment for less than $500. Nothing matched and it didn't matter. I was happy as a clam. The monthly rent was about $400.

A few years after Maureen and I were married, our building was converted to a co-operative corporation, which resulted in favorable prices for those of us who were renters. We purchased my little junior-sized apartment and, as the years went by, moved to a larger, two-bedroom apartment where the boys were raised. We had a bunk bed with a pull-out trundle bed in a drawer, and that's where all three slept: Josh, the oldest, was on top; Luke, next in line, was in the middle; and Jake, the baby, was on the trundle, closest to the floor, so there would be no danger if he fell out. They all loved the arrangement. Just as Josh was entering high school, the neighbor's studio apartment became available and we connected it to ours, giving Josh his own bedroom and bath.

The building entrance at 525 East 86 Street is flush with the sidewalk and located just half a block from Carl Schurz Park. The park contains the building and grounds of Gracie Mansion, the Mayor's official residence; a three-block-long promenade overlooking the East River; and a large playground area for young children that has swings, slipper slides, monkey bars for climbing, sandboxes and water sprinkler. When our boys were growing up, a daily trip to the park was a must, and there Maureen met and made lifelong friendships with several other mothers who had children the same age as our own.

Both the building and the park are easily accessible to a wheelchair. Nowadays, in warm weather I spend an hour or more in the park almost every day, enjoying river traffic, a basketball pickup game by local youths or small dogs romping in the puppy run situated adjacent to the promenade.

LAW PRACTICES

During my 40 years practicing law, considerable changes took place not only in our firm and the manner in which we operated but also in the interpretation of patent law itself.

When I arrived at Morgan, Finnegan, Durham and Pine in 1963, the firm had fewer than 20 lawyers. Ten years later, I became the twelfth partner in the firm's history. By 2003, when I retired, the firm —now called Morgan & Finnegan—had more than 30 partners and nearly 100 lawyers as well as branch offices in Washington, D.C. and San Francisco.

The patent law business in the 1960s was carried out very differently from the way it is today. There were no computers in those days, no instant copy machines, no telephone facsimile machines, no email transmissions, no computer searching services, and no cell phones or text messaging.

Back then, secretaries used carbon paper to produce a maximum of five or six copies of a document, and they literally had to pound the keys on their manual typewriters so that all copies were legible. To issue a large number of copies, we used a mimeograph machine. You'd type the original, put it on a drum, and crank out multiple inked copies. To make a copy of an existing document, we used a machine called a *thermofax,* which did *wet* copying. Copies were submerged in a bath, and they had to dry before they could be handed around. A telex machine that produced messages similar to a telegram was the only quick way to correspond with an overseas office; the second quickest was a courier service. Sometimes packages were handed to the airplane pilot who would personally make the delivery. Briefs submitted to appellate courts were printed and bound by specialty printing companies. Case law research was carried out by laboriously reading through digests of *head notes* of legal principles decided in reported decisions.

While legal work today is much faster and perhaps more efficient, the end product seems to have diminished in the process. Writing lacks finesse, color and nuance. I see fewer clever turns of phrase or elegantly constructed sentences and paragraphs in correspondence among lawyers or in case law decisions. With computer-generated email messages, letters and briefs, speed matters more than carefully considered use of language.

The most thoughtfully written treatise on the subject of my specialty, patent law, is still the 1890 three-volume work, *Robinson On Patents*, that was written by a professor at Yale University. Case law decisions written in the late 1800s through the 1950s reflect careful attention to every fact and detail, all referenced and annotated with the applicable legal principles by a thorough and compelling analysis. In comparing those earlier decisions to the decisions written in recent years, I can only wonder how the judges found the time to craft such lengthy and masterful expositions of law and fact.

In patent law practice, the Achilles' heel for the putative inventor has always been the requirement that the subject matter of the invention must not have been obvious to the person of ordinary skill working in the art at the time the alleged invention was made. During my first 20 years in the profession, there was no consistency in the courts' rulings on the pivotal question of *obviousness*. Lawyers arguing for the inventor attempted to use testimony and documentation to show that workers in the *art* of the invention were baffled by a problem which the inventor had solved. Proving the old adage that *everything is obvious in hindsight*, too often once the trial court judges or the appellate court judges were schooled in the subject of the invention, they would put themselves in the shoes of the workers in the art and conclude that the invention would have been obvious at the time made. As a result, they would strike down the patent.

In an attempt to prevent inconsistency in patent rulings and give the business world incentive to continue to invest in research and innovation, Congress created a new court of appeals to hear all patent case appeals in 1982. For the next 25 years of my career, the patent appeals court developed a set of objective tests that required a court to rule that the invention under consideration would not have been obvious to ordinary workers in the art at the time made—regardless of the judge's own subjective view. As a result, inventors found more *teeth* in their patented advances; damage awards for infringement increased; and both individuals and corporate manufacturers were encouraged to invest time and money in research.

From 1982 until my retirement, the patent system was alive and well, flourishing even. Once more, I was lucky, being able to play my small part in the patent world during a time when lawyers' efforts on behalf of inventors were richly rewarding and there was an atmosphere of respect for inventors.

Subsequent to my retirement, the U.S. Supreme Court unfortunately struck down a patent in 2007, ruling that, despite the findings of non-obviousness by objective tests, workers in the art eventually would have made the invention in question; and that it was only a matter of time before the inventor's work would have been discovered by others. Sadly, the Court's justices looked into their own crystal ball to predict the future, thereby erasing 25 years of work by the specialty patent appeals court.

It is now up to Congress to enact new patent legislation, setting out specific objective factual tests which must be considered in the determination of the obvious/non-obvious issue. These might include: commercial success (independent of marketing/sales prowess); copying by others in the industry; a long-felt need in the art for a *better way* to accomplish a result; the failure of others who tried to solve the same problem; or the spawning of further advances or improvements in the industry based upon the inventor's discovery.

The legislation should further provide that when two or more of these objective facts are found to exist, it is mandatory upon the court to hold that the invention was not obvious to persons of ordinary skill in the art at the time made.

Only time will tell, but I believe that if Congress is willing to follow through on its creation of the specialty appeals court for patents; it will pass such legislation forthwith.

LIGHTER MOMENTS

Patent law practice is serious business. There might be millions of dollars at stake in soliciting or defending a patented invention. One casual misstep or misstatement by a lawyer might mean losing the patent rights and the client as well. In such a tense situation, light moments were especially welcome and long remembered.

One that I recall dates back to the period after the firm's first large Xerox copier arrived. I spotted a fellow from the office next door rummaging through his secretary's wastebasket after 5 p.m., just after she'd left for the day. I thought nothing of it until I spotted him doing the same thing, at the same time, the following day.

"John," I couldn't help but ask, "What are you looking for?"

"I'm making sure there are no original papers in here."

"Why would original papers be in a waste basket?"

"Because," he explained, "Yesterday, I asked my secretary to make a copy of a paper. She came back with the copy but not the original. When I asked for it, she said, 'Oh, I thought you wanted just the copy. I threw the original away." He sighed, exasperated. "Now, I don't trust her."

Back then, the policy at the firm was to maintain a certain formality. Staff members were supposed to address attorneys— only males, at that time— as "Mr."

One day, a new receptionist was answering the phones. At one point, the intercom sounded: "HarrEE, your mother's on the phone!" A new member of our office, Harry Marcus, got no end of ribbing for this one.

In the early 1970s, I was working on a case pending in the California district court in Los Angeles and was scheduled to present an argument before the judge handling the case. It would be my first appearance, and I wanted to make a good impression. Since my hair had grown a bit long I made sure to get a trim before I left home.

I was in court when the bailiff announced the judge's entry. In came Judge Whelan, sporting long, shaggy, nearly shoulder-length curls. I had had nothing to worry about.

In another case in the 1970s, pending in New York's own Southern District Court before Judge Constance Baker Motley (recently appointed based on her work arguing Civil Rights cases before the Supreme Court in the 1960s), the parties were ordered to have a sort of mini-trial on the single issue of obviousness—always the *sticky wicket*. In this case, our firm was against the patent, so the opposing side was first up.

Judge Motley surveyed the assembled attorneys and the array of file cabinets, storage boxes and papers spread on the tables. "Gentlemen," she exclaimed, "We're here on a single, tiny issue for a very short trial. What are all these materials? I don't see how we'll get to all this stuff!"

The judge obviously had a far different view of the proofs required to establish the pro or con of the obviousness issue than we lawyers, fighting vigorously for our clients. But the tide soon turned favorably for our side.

The opposition was adducing testimony from its expert witness regarding the teachings and scope of its patent. Then, abruptly, the plaintiff's attorney announced, "Your Honor, that completes this witness's testimony on this subject, but he will be back next week to testify on defendant's prior art contentions."

Judge Motley was taken aback. "Counselor, this case will be over by Friday. There will be no next week. If this witness has more to say, he'd better say it now."

A bit flustered, the opposing attorney had no choice but to launch into the pieces of drawings and articles we had identified, as showing there was nothing new in the patent drawings. Shortly afterward, the attorney showed his expert witness our best prior art drawing. Immediately, the opposing witness stated emphatically, "*Now* you make a better case for obviousness!"

At the same moment that I very quietly remarked on this damaging statement to my colleague, Judge Motley turned to our table, "Did you hear that, did you hear that? He said the patent was obvious!"

Needless to say, we won the case. Never again did an opposing expert witness support our side of a case with such finality. Adding insult to injury, the opposing attorney's wallet was stolen the last day of our brief trial. I'm afraid this story was not so humorous to him.

In the mid-80s, our firm brought a patent action against a large corporation for alleged infringement of our client's invention relating to a hip prosthesis—an artificial hip implant.

The defendant counterclaimed, alleging that our client had infringed on a patent that had been issued several years earlier. When I did my research—in *Robinson On Patents*, of course—I learned that a patent owner might be stopped from enforcing the patent if there has been "open and notorious" infringement for a number of years without action. The rationale for this doctrine is that the accused infringer has relied on the patentee's inaction and that therefore it is not equitable for the patent owner to reap a benefit from its misleading conduct.

After marshalling all the evidence, we moved for a summary judgment that the infringer's patent was unenforceable. The case was tried before District Judge Maryanne Trump Barry (sister of real estate developer Donald Trump). In the course of oral argument on the issue, Judge Barry commented to our side, "So, counsel, you're saying that this patent holder was waiting for the grape to get ripe enough to pluck?"

With that, the opposing counsel jumped out of his chair, unable to restrain himself, virtually shouting. "Your Honor, you make it sound like my client was lying in the weeds!" He was simultaneously pleading and indignant.

"Counsel," replied the judge. "That's exactly what I meant to say!"

A few weeks later, Judge Barry filed her decision, granting summary judgment holding the defendant's patent unenforceable. The exchange between Judge Barry and defendant's attorney in court had said it all. It is simply unfair for a patent holder to remain silent while another person, relying on that silence, builds up a business, and for the patent holder then to strike like a snake or a stalking cat—bringing a patent infringement suit that seeks damages for sales already made as well as an injunction against further sales.

From my point of view, it was a most satisfying result, demonstrating the success that can be achieved when a lawyer pursues each aspect of his or her work: researching diligently, marshalling the evidence in detail, briefing the court, and successfully defending the rationale for the controlling principle of law.

COURTROOM DRAMAS

Patent law practice is often considered an arcane area, the domain of eccentric inventors and *stuffed shirt* lawyers who make their points using esoteric scientific terminology in excruciating detail. But I have found patent litigation to offer its own Perry Mason moments, with suspenseful buildups, dirty dealing, even last-minute courtroom revelations. Here are a few.

The Case of the Indented Document

In patent law, it is often critical that the inventor establish the exact date on which the invention was conceived. That becomes the cut-off date for determining the level and extent of knowledge possessed by the average person working in the field at the time the invention was made.

Our client was the accused infringer in a case where the patent related to the type of electrical outlet boxes that are mounted inside the wall and hold the outlet receptacle into which an appliance is plugged. During the pretrial exchange of contentions and documents, the inventor committed himself to a specific date on which he had conceived his invention.

My firm had asked that the purported inventor submit

all the documents in his personal files regarding his putative invention. Among them was a three- or four-page brochure. During pretrial interrogation, the inventor had contended that the brochure came into his hands sometime after he conceived and developed his patented outlet box. This was a critical piece of testimony because the outlet box illustrated in the brochure was remarkably similar to the outlet box described in the patent. The brochure was undated and the company that issued it was no longer in business, so it seemed we would not be able to ascertain the publication date.

Shortly before the scheduled trial, I picked up the brochure and was about to turn to the inside pages when indentations on the cover page caught my eye. I studied the page briefly, angling the brochure to the light and trying to catch the shadows created by the indentations, and I began to make out what seemed to be the inventor's signature. I handed the brochure to my secretary. "See if the guys in the copying room can make a Xerox that shows up the indented writing on the cover page."

To my amazement, they produced a copy that clearly showed notes about a telephone message, dated and signed in the inventor's handwriting. And then came the real payoff. When I checked the date of the telephone conversation, I discovered that the indented date written on the brochure was prior to the inventor's claimed date of conception.

In the space of some 15 minutes, I realized I had broken the case wide open. Obviously, the brochure was on the inventor's desk when he had the telephone conversation and was underneath the sheet of memo paper on which he wrote his name and the date. Instead of designing a new and novel outlet box, the putative inventor had merely made minor modifications to the box illustrated in the brochure.

The plaintiff had requested a jury trial—relatively rare at the time—so we decided to hold our discovery quiet until after the inventor had appeared on the stand. Sure enough, he testified about the magnitude of his advance in the world of outlet boxes. In our defense, we called a retired NYPD detective who explained to the jury how police used a special lamp, called a *half-light*, to examine indented documents.

The courtroom lights were lowered and, as the jurors gathered around the lamp, murmuring excitedly, the detective then turned on the half-light over the brochure and read aloud the date and the inventor's signature. Several members of the jury exclaimed, "Yes, I see it too!"

The jury found the plaintiff's patent invalid, and the court ultimately awarded a portion of our attorney fees to our client. We had turned this patent infringement trial into a trial of veracity and the jury had no difficulty finding the inventor's testimony untruthful or, at least, unreliable.

The Case of the Chinese Fingers Invention

I spent the majority of my time from 1985 through 2000 defending the patent rights of our client in the field of artificial hip implant devices. Broken or arthritic hip joints are commonplace throughout the world, so many readers will be familiar with hip replacement surgery and the wonderful relief from pain a prosthetic hip affords.

The first of these implants were solid metallic pieces with a stem that was inserted in the canal of the patient's femur bone and a large ball head that fitted into the acetabulum (cup) of the hip saddle bone. These devices remain viable today, particularly for elderly patients with a broken femur head. However, in younger, active patients, the solid ball head is undesirable since it soon wears a hole in the bone of the acetabulum.

The next advance in this field was a two-part device, a metal-backed cup that fit snugly into the acetabulum. Its interior was filled with a rigid plastic liner, and a much smaller ball head of the stem was friction-fitted into it. These devices eliminated wear on the acetabular bone, but the friction-fit proved unreliable and resulted in many hip dislocations.

The challenge was to find a way to lock the ball head to the rigid plastic interior lining of the cup, yet allow the surgeon freedom to easily unlock and re-lock the two parts together during surgery, when he is working in a pool of blood.

Our client's solution was to hollow out an interior space in the rigid plastic liner with an annular (ring-shaped), sloping outer wall and a separate internal locking ring that could slide up and down in the interior space. The outside wall of the sliding ring is sloped to match the sloping wall of the plastic liner. The inner diameter of the locking ring allows the ball head to slip through only when the ring is pushed up to the top of its sliding space; once the ball head is fully inserted, the locking ring slips back down behind the maximum diameter of the ball. Any further attempt to remove the ball head is fruitless. The greater the force tending to pull out the ball head, the greater the gripping action of the locking ring against the sloped wall of the cup's interior space.

The *key* to unlock the parts was a small half-circle annular projecting ring inserted around the ball head of the stem. The key pushes up the locking ring, once again allowing the ball head to be easily removed from the cup member.

Our client's patented hip prosthesis was, and remains to this day, a huge commercial success. A large corporate competitor in the industry soon copied it. Our infringement suit quickly followed. However, pretrial *discovery* procedures were complicated and time-consuming, as the infringer pulled out all stops in an effort to raise some technical defense to the patent. About two years later, I learned that one of the defendant's employees who had worked on the design of the product accused to infringe was now working elsewhere in the industry.

I telephoned him and gingerly broached the subject of the litigation and his part in the development of the product in question. If he would give favorable testimony, I could take his deposition and it would become part of the trial evidence. After a few minutes, he finally said, "I'm not going to volunteer anything. But if you ask the right questions I'll give you the right answers."

That was enough for me. He was located in the Midwest, so we agreed on Chicago for the deposition. Still, I was a bit worried as to the outcome, since at one point in our telephone conversation he had said he was surprised at the similarity between the accused product and our client's product.

As the questioning progressed, it took the following turn:

Q. What, if anything, did you have in front of you when you set out to design your company's hip implant device?

A. Well, I had never seen any part used as a key, and after we manufactured our key, I was quite surprised at how similar the products were.

Q. You're talking about the little key for unlocking the ball head from the cup, correct?

A. Yes. I had never seen it before.

Q. How about the locking ring itself, which could slide inside the cup, between locked and unlocked positions? How did you arrive at that configuration?

A. Oh. That. Well, I saw the plaintiff's product. It works like the Chinese Fingers trap: the harder you pull, the tighter it gets. I wouldn't have thought of that in a hundred years!

I hadn't expected this witness to be so expressive or so laudatory of the patented invention. The testimony coming from the defendant's own product designer sealed the case for our client. In the settlement that followed shortly, our client received a multi-million dollar payment.

The Case of the Intimidated Witness

We often hear of indicted criminal defendants attempting to bribe a jury member or intimidating a potential witness. That happened to our client in a patent case.

The patented invention covered an immunoassay, a test for detecting disease—in this case, a test to detect the hepatitis B virus. Our firm was defending the accused infringer, and our expert witness was an immunologist practicing and performing research at the Mayo Clinic in Rochester, Minnesota. The evening before our expert was scheduled to testify, the hotel clerk handed me a telephone message from the Mayo Clinic to pass on to him. Later that evening, our expert mentioned that the party we were opposing had advised his superiors that he was about to give testimony that might reflect negatively on the institution.

The next day we put our expert on the stand. When we asked him to recount the gist of the conversation he had told us about, the courtroom was hushed—and then we asked if that conversation would affect his testimony. With obvious deep emotion and conviction, our doctor testified that he still remembered how honored he had felt that first day of his tenure at the world-renowned institution, and that the idea that he would ever do anything to besmirch the reputation of his revered hospital was absolutely unthinkable.

Our witness then gave his testimony, never wavering from the position he had taken in the written reports he had provided to the opposing party.

The judge ruled in our favor, saying his decision was based on a technical defect in the patent's description of the invention's advance over previously known techniques. But I remain convinced the decision was prompted, in part, on the patent owner's scurrilous conduct.

The Case of the Missing Sketch

This case involved a much-needed solution to the problem of *thigh pain* experienced by a small number of patients who had received an artificial hip implant. It seems that these individuals had unusually enlarged canals in their femur bones that caused the end tip of the implant's metal stem to move slightly and create a pressure point on the femur bone.

Our client was the patent holder. His patent included a series of cylindrical end tips (sleeves) with varying outer diameters that could be attached to the end of the prosthetic stem, allowing the surgeon to match the prosthesis to both the acetabulum and the femur canal during the replacement surgery.

The attorney for the defendant called to the stand an ex-employee who testified that he had thought of the same solution and actually sketched it out on a piece of paper while sitting with a fellow worker at his kitchen table. Although this witness testified that he had had the idea long before our client, he admitted he no longer had the piece of paper and that there was no other written record that might serve to corroborate his testimony.

As we began our cross-examination, the judge noted that the day was nearly over and asked that we be brief so the witness could return home quickly. Thus, he had made it clear that he had no intention of giving any weight or credence to such self-serving, uncorroborated "recollections."

INVENTORS

I never had a boring day in my 40 years of patent law practice, thanks to the wide variety of technology that came across my desk, the fact that every patent or application for a patent involved something believed to be new, and the particular issues of patent law raised by the making of each invention. What also kept things interesting were the unique personalities and areas of expertise of the inventors.

Drawing up an application for a patent often involves several face-to-face meetings with the inventor and innumerable telephone conversations. It requires a careful, detailed, word-for-word analysis of the prior works or methods, a thorough description of the invention for which the patent is sought, and an explanation of how the invention differs from whatever preceded it.

During the process, I often became a confidante of sorts to my inventor clients, who were as a group intelligent, curious and, most significantly, keenly observant of their surroundings.

That's what makes them special. Most people don't even look at what's in front of them. Others look, but don't see. An inventor's curiosity leads him to ask questions: "What's going on here? Why does it happen? How does it work? Is there a better way? Could I use this idea in another application?"

The rest of us ask only, "Why didn't I think of that?"

The fastening product Velcro best demonstrates this phenomenon. Invented in the middle of the twentieth century, it has become one of the most commercially successful patented products the world has ever known.

Velcro involves a combination of two strips of material, one with a multitude of tiny, flexible hooks and the other with an equal number of tiny, flexible hoops. When the strips are pressed together, eureka! The materials lock together. To be separated, they must be forcibly peeled apart.

For centuries, every farmer, hiker or cowhand has noticed how sand burrs stick tenaciously to your pant legs when you're walking or riding through underbrush. When I was a youngster on the farm, nearly every day several burrs stuck to my pants and shoelaces. In picking them off, I'd often prick my finger on one of the tiny, sharp hooks on the rounded surface of the sand burr. (You can see them if you look carefully.) These hooks embed themselves into the threaded loops of woven pants fabric, which is why they're so hard to pry off.

The Velcro strips work in just the same way. George de Mestral, a Swiss mountaineer and inventor, observed the hook-and-loop phenomenon when his dog was covered with burrs after a walk on a summer day in 1948. De Mestral examined one under a microscope and was inspired to adapt the idea to a fastening system.

(Now, why didn't I think of that?)

One of my clients, Eugeniusz (Gene) Rylewski, a mechanical engineer, was similarly inspired. He was trying to solve the problem of cavitation in water pumps. That's the phenomenon whereby cavities—vapor bubbles—are formed, as fluid on the low-pressure suction side flows over impeller blades. These cavities collapse rapidly, causing shock waves that pit the surface of the blade and thus ultimately cause the pump to fail.

The cavitation action emits a loud, crackling noise because the collapsing liquid moves faster than the speed of sound. Knowing that, Gene realized that fluid's flow over an impeller blade is analogous to airflow over the wing of an aircraft. The *lift* provided by the wing is, in fact, a vacuum or low-pressure area, created by the shape of the wing. Gene incorporated various aerodynamic elements in his designs for fluid-handling machines.

As a result, he was able to reduce surge fluctuations, mechanical vibrations and noise levels, and to delay significantly the onset of cavitation in water pumps and similar devices. Gene's observation of the analogy led to his receipt of numerous patents.

Like other inventors I have known, Gene was always mentally sifting through information to cull out whatever might be useful. He was fluent in Russian, German and French in addition to English and his native Polish, and he sought out Russian and German physics and engineering textbooks, which he said disclosed problems and solutions most explicitly.

Once, Gene had a Friday meeting with a client who mentioned that several issues had them stumped. Recalling a solution to the problem in one of his Russian textbooks, he spent a carefree couple of days skiing but came in on Monday morning with the solution to his client's problems. The client greatly appreciated his diligent *work* over the weekend.

I have the greatest respect for my inventor clients, though sometimes they leave me a little bemused.

I worked with Sanford Redmond for a number of years on machinery for automatically producing butter pats at the rate of 1500 per minute. He also developed machinery and new designs for single-use dispensing packages, creamer packages and various other tubes and containers. His machinery designs seemed to follow one cardinal rule: never use reciprocating parts—that is, parts that work together with one another in a back-and-forth motion—because they inevitably wear out and fall apart. Everything in Redmond's machines rotates; the material is continuously conveyed from one rotating forming operation to another. Sandy has been granted nearly 30 patents in this country and hundreds of counterpart (equivalent) patents throughout the world.

While Sandy's machines are impeccably designed, he would often draw freehand sketches of his next idea as we worked together. I never got much out of looking at those sketches, which were often crudely drawn and incorporated several views in one. Sandy had worked out his ideas in his own mind, but he couldn't produce them in a single, comprehensible drawing.

Choose life, that thou mayest live ...
Deuteronomy 30:19

Part Three: Living with ALS

SIGNS

Someone who isn't working in the field of patent litigation probably does not realize the degree of physical and mental stress involved. Almost all the cases are complex, and mastering all the aspects of each litigated issue takes long hours of concentrated study and the quality attributed to Winston Churchill—*an elephantine memory*.

The work is so demanding and all-engrossing that you may focus on it to the exclusion of other concerns. I suppose that's why it was so easy for me to ignore the initial sign that something was wrong with my body and then to continue to ignore successive signs for several years thereafter.

The first inklings came in 1993. I had already spent three years of intense and continuous involvement in two major and complex cases, neither of which would be resolved until 2001. Tens of millions of dollars were at stake for the litigants in each. The pretrial, trial and appeal phases were more or less simultaneous, though one trial took place from 1993 to 1995 and the other from late 1996 through mid-1997.

To dig out the facts means poring over and becoming thoroughly familiar with hundreds of documents as well as with a dozen or two deposition transcripts, several expert-witness reports and other written pretrial responses. I had also to master all the relevant legal precedent.

Before the trial, each party is required to file briefs on the law and proposed findings of facts which they plan to establish (i.e. prove) from documents and witness testimony to be introduced into evidence at the trial. Extensive preparation is needed to elicit positive testimony from friendly witnesses and to cross-examine the opposition effectively. When the trial is in progress, I had to prepare numerous legal memoranda on the evidentiary issues that arise. And after the trials, both cases required post-trial and appellate briefs, exhaustively annotated to the trial evidence of record.

Also, a lot of travel was involved. Relevant documents, witnesses and courtrooms were overseas in England (London and Southampton), Munich (where the European Patent Office is located), and Strasbourg (home of the World Court of Human Rights). In the U.S., they were in Chicago, Los Angeles, Louisville, St. Louis, Memphis, Palm Beach and St. Petersburg, Florida and Warsaw, Indiana.

In the summer of 1993, when the first trial was starting, I noticed that if I sat in one position for two or three hours, I needed a couple of moments to muster the strength to change position and a few more to stand. Since I had been hunched over my desk for hours on end over a period of several months, I didn't pay much attention to this fleeting weakness. I attributed it to the trial-preparation work.

From 1993 to 1995, I had occasional bouts of unusual stiffness in my upper body and some leg fatigue. I dismissed these problems as well, attributing them to the stress of dealing with one trial while doing final pretrial work on the other.

Then, in September 1995, after a court appearance on a post-trial motion in the first of the cases, I was late for a flight. I was startled to find that I was unable to run through the airport corridors but could manage only a sort of half-trot. I missed the flight by less than ten minutes. Though I was puzzled to find I'd apparently lost some of the strength in my legs, again I brushed off the symptom as merely a sign of fatigue or insufficient physical activity.

At about the same time, carrying my briefcase had become difficult, so I switched to one with a shoulder strap. And when I walked, I felt that my shoulders were being pulled forward into a stoop, so I kept my hands in my trouser pockets, pressing against my thighs to keep myself upright.

Though I probably mentioned these issues to Maureen, I said nothing to anyone else. I considered them only minor distractions. And no one else seemed to take notice of them.

By the summer of 1996, however, I could no longer walk at a normal gait. I had to move my legs more slowly and deliberately, and I became fatigued after walking only three or four blocks. I went on a business trip to London at the time, bringing along my older son, Josh, as a college graduation treat. I vividly recall walking alongside him and repeatedly asking him to please slow down as I couldn't keep up with his pace.

That fall, I no longer could ignore the fact that my leg and stomach muscles were continuing to weaken. At Maureen's insistence, in November 1996 I went to see a neurologist friend, Gerald Silverman. He diagnosed my problem as adult onset progressive spinal muscular atrophy (SMA) caused by a recessive genetic defect, and warned me that the weakness in my legs would escalate. But he put the situation in the best light possible. He advised that the disease was not life-threatening and suggested that walking with a cane was actually a "look of distinction."

At the time, I didn't fully appreciate the seriousness of Doctor Silverman's diagnosis. I think that as a friend, he didn't want to frighten me unnecessarily since it was likely the weakness would progress very slowly. I was still focused on the trial for my second case, which was scheduled to begin in early December, slightly more than two weeks away. But I did check some medical textbooks. They confirmed that for adult patients with SMA, muscle deterioration was, indeed, very slow, occurring "over decades." I found no cross-reference to ALS, but thought it odd that newborns with SMA rarely survived more than 12 to18 months, while adults lived on for years. I concluded that time was on my side and that while I might grow somewhat weaker, nothing much would change for many years to come.

In the next few months and into the early summer of 1997, coping with the fatigue in my legs and mid-section had become increasingly difficult. Meanwhile, the trial dragged on and involved numerous trips from New York to Louisville. The trial sessions lasted for two- or three-week periods, with a month's break in between.

By then, even the trips back and forth to the courthouse had become a physical challenge to me. Air travel—involving briefcases, clothing bags and long walks through airport terminals—was exhausting. As the weeks of the trial turned into months, the muscles in my legs and stomach continued to deteriorate at an accelerating pace.

By the end of the trial in April 1997, I was unable to walk a full block without resting. Though I didn't need support, each step felt precarious, as if my legs might give way at any moment. During the last days of the trial, our team of lawyers was lunching in a cafeteria when I discovered I could no longer carry a food tray while I walked. Holding an umbrella over my head also became impossible. In the shower, I could not lift my arms over my head to wash my hair. Soon, I showered sitting on a chair.

Through all of these setbacks, I was able to keep a stoic attitude—*a stiff upper lip*, so to speak— telling myself that I still had many years to live and that walking with a cane wouldn't be the worst thing in the world. Though I could no longer pretend to my trial colleagues that all was normal, I reassured them that my difficulties were most likely hereditary and certainly not contagious.

Shortly afterwards, during that summer of 1997, the wall of denial I had put up began to crack. Maureen and I had gone to our corner diner for breakfast. Although it was less than a half block away, I could barely make the effort to take the last few steps, and I virtually collapsed into the chair. I looked across the table to Maureen. She didn't have to say a word. Her expression was sympathetic and her eyes were full of sadness. In that moment, we both acknowledged that the comfortable existence we had led was no longer to be.

Tears welled up in my eyes and then spilled down my cheeks. Maureen took my hands. Weeping quietly, we sat for several minutes. I continued my struggle to stop the tears and stifle the quiver in my lips and chin.

Maureen spoke first. "Bob, we just have to get through this somehow. I love you, and I'm not going anywhere. We'll find a way. I know we will."

At that moment, we both acknowledged it was unlikely that I could anticipate merely a slow decline in my faculties over the next twenty or thirty years. In less than a year, I had already experienced a dramatic loss of strength in my stomach muscles and both my legs.

We had to know what lay ahead.

ADJUSTMENTS

We met with more doctors and I had more tests: a muscle biopsy, an MRI, an EMG, a second EKG, and then a spinal tap. I received second, third and fourth opinions. By the fall of 1997, my diagnosis had become clearer. I had Amyotrophic Lateral Sclerosis (ALS), a motor neutron disease that was first described in 1869 by French neurologist Jean-Martin Charcot. It's commonly known in the U.S. as Lou Gehrig's disease, after the famous Yankee ballplayer who was its best-known victim. (He retired when he was diagnosed in 1939.)

I was being treated, in fact, at Columbia University Hospital's Lou Gehrig ALS Center when we first began to comprehend my situation. Maureen had casually inquired of a clinical nurse what we could expect regarding the course of the disease. The nurse was brutally frank.

"Your husband will first lose all function in his legs and then in his arms and hands. Next, he won't be able to swallow. Finally, his lungs won't function and he'll die of respiratory failure." In response to Maureen's shocked expression, she added—as if this made it better—"Of course, in the end, we all die of respiratory failure."

We left her office abruptly. Now it was Maureen who

couldn't hold back the tears.

I began to try various measures to help me get to and from work. First, I used a cane. This helped me walk from my apartment elevator to a car waiting at the street curb and from the street directly into my office building. That worked for perhaps three months, but then one day my knees buckled and I crumpled to the floor of our apartment building's lobby.

Then I used a lightweight, fold-up wheelchair. Maureen would roll me from the apartment to our car or a taxi, and the building doorman would help me transfer into the car. When we were near the office, I'd phone my secretary and she'd meet the car accompanied by an office clerk who volunteered to help me out of the car, into the wheelchair, and then into my office chair. We reversed the process on the trip home. We kept up this routine for a year or so.

At the time, Josh worked in an office near mine, and several times a week he assisted with the evening transfer from office chair to the car. At noontime, my nephew Will, the husband of my niece Jenni, came to my office to walk me to the bathroom and help me urinate. I had to be very careful with fluid intake so I could wait until Will arrived. In the bathroom, Will hoisted me onto a high stool so I could sit while I urinated, since it was impossible for me to remain standing.

At least my hands and arms remained unaffected during both trials and appellate hearings, so working wasn't a problem, but within two years I could not use them either.

The emotional impact of the gradual loss of my abilities was overwhelming. Eventually, I could not hold my hand steady enough to insert my contact lenses. Constipation became an issue, but if I overmedicated even slightly, I'd have the opposite problem. I'd need assistance from Maureen or my sons just to get to the toilet or to clean myself. As each type of movement became more difficult or was lost forever, I had more crying jags—mostly private ones.

One Saturday morning, Maureen and I had driven to a bakery in Greenwich Village renowned for its doughnuts. When Maureen brought the bag of doughnuts to the car, I discovered I couldn't raise my hands to my mouth even to take a bite. That was only a small disappointment, but added to the mounting list of my disabilities and losses, it sent me into despair. I could only sit back and sob.

Fortunately, I managed to find some occasional humor in my plight. In a magazine for people with disabilities, I had found an ad for a spring-loaded seat cushion that delivered a boost to someone having difficulty rising from a chair. I had bought one and was sitting on it one morning when I absent mindedly leaned over to tie my shoestrings. The cushion went into action, jettisoning me right onto my head. As I lay sprawled on the floor, I could only laugh at my ridiculous predicament.

On another occasion I had just thanked profusely one of the young men in the office who helped me from the wheelchair to a taxi. He shrugged it off. "Don't worry, Mr. Paulson. I'm used to lifting dead weight. I work in a mortuary on weekends." The fellow was sincerely trying to make me feel comfortable, but his awkwardly expressed statement struck my funny bone.

As I thought to myself, "I may be dead weight, but I'm not quite ready for the mortician."

I was still working long hours at this time. I often went into to my office on Sundays, when the escalators weren't in service all the way to the lower lobby level. Reaching them meant a long, slow ascent up a flight of stairs as I used the railing to pull myself up.

One Sunday, the building porter on duty saw me come through the door and head for the stairway. He asked me to wait a moment, and then he disappeared. A moment later, the escalator started running. I hadn't thought to ask if that was possible, but the man had obviously observed me and decided to help. His gesture was among the nicest I have received from any stranger who observed my disability.

During this time, when I was at home in the evenings and needed help being lifted from the wheelchair to a desk chair, couch, bathroom or bed, I relied primarily on Jake, the youngest of my sons and the only one then still living with us. Though he was only 15 or 16, Jake was exceptionally willing to help. Although my situation was especially hard for him to accept in the teenage years, his reassuring presence made him one of my strongest pillars of support. Josh was living only a short distance away, and he, too, never hesitated to come over and help give me a lift. Luke, who was attending college in Colorado at the time, took over the lifting during school breaks. I would have been lost without their unfailing love and strong backs.

I appreciated also the times when my family could poke a little fun at me. Once, for example, I remarked to the boys that my arms and legs were wasting away to the point that I soon would resemble Stick Man—the kind of figure young children draw to represent their fathers. "No," one said in response. "We think *Floppy Poppy* is more like it."

Their mother, Maureen, came up with an especially outrageous idea. It was nearing Halloween, and in Greenwich Village the neighborhood artists, bohemians, and individualists of every sexual persuasion celebrate the chance for self-expression with a spectacular parade—what the website describes as "hundreds of puppets, 53 Bands of different types of Musicians, Dancers and Artists, and thousands of other New Yorkers in Costumes of Their Own Creation in the Nation's Most Wildly Creative Public Participatory Event!" Even with all the capital letters, that's an understatement.

The sidewalks overflow with masked and costumed (and often barely costumed) spectators and paraders. Many restaurants get into the spirit of the occasion by putting up decorations and presenting their waitstaff in costumes. One such was Fujiyama Mama; our friends Mike and Susan often invited us to join them there for dinner to enjoy the festivities.

It was my first Halloween in a wheelchair, and Maureen's inspiration was that I should dress as the victim of a bad accident. I agreed that was the perfect costume. So she fashioned an arm sling from a pillowcase, wrapped rolls of gauze around my head and one leg, and borrowed scar-like decals from a neighbor's four-year-old to stick on my cheek. She herself donned a nun's costume and called herself "Sister Mary, Quite Contrary." At the restaurant, other diners regarded me quizzically, as if wondering if I truly had broken bones. "They have no idea that I'm actually worse off than I look," I said to my group.

On their way out, a family with a young boy passed by our table and gave me a long once-over. A moment later, the father popped back inside and came over to me. "I have no idea if you're for real or not," he said. "But either way, you've got a helluva sense of humor!" That was the perfect capper to the evening.

VIEW FROM A WHEELCHAIR

In about the middle of 1998, the fragile routine I'd established with volunteer helpers came undone and I had a rude awakening to the facts of life in the world of the disabled.

The young office workers who were helping to lift me became worried about dropping me or injuring their backs. Since assisting me was not within the staffers' job descriptions, the firm was concerned that if one was injured in the course of helping me, it could be vulnerable to a lawsuit for medical expenses. One of the doormen at my building began to balk at helping as I became weaker and harder to lift and maneuver into a car. And then there was a last straw: My secretary of more than 15 years abruptly announced she could no longer work for me, as my physical weakness and the sight of the wheelchair in the office were simply "too depressing."

When I heard this, I asked that my secretary leave the firm. I didn't want to hear her name or see her face again. I regarded her behavior as an act of desertion at a time when I needed her most. Despite my dismay, the firm allowed her to stay, simply moving her to a desk on the other side of the office floor. The attitude seemed to be *business as usual*.

The unspoken but very clear message was, "Figure out a way to take care of yourself Bob, and find a new secretary. The firm can make good use of the one you've trained so well."

The departure of someone on whom I had relied for so many years and the lack of support from the firm were demeaning and humiliating blows. Though I'd been a partner at the place for thirty years, I now felt like a pariah. That wasn't all. After I became ill, every year the firm proposed additional cuts in my percentage interest in its income. Since I was in a wheelchair, it seemed, *ipso facto* my worth to the firm had diminished. Yet each year, an examination of the records showed that I was still among the six or seven highest-billing partners. The suggestion was withdrawn.

Once I was forever confined to my wheelchair, I realized that my perspective would be altered in every way. I'd have to deal not only with my physical problems but also with the struggle to maintain my self-esteem and sense of worth. And, no small thing, I'd have to overcome the constant embarrassment and self-consciousness of being unable to move around on my own.

SINGING

Eventually, ALS took away my ability to sing. That was a very hard blow to absorb. I had found singing especially rewarding, when I was in high school, and it continued to give me pleasure through my college years and well into my adult life.

At K-State I had become a member of the first Men's Varsity Glee Club, organized in 1957 by music professor Morris Hays. Professor Hays was the ideal director for a men's chorus— always cheerful, full of energy and enthusiasm, and very much at ease in getting a bunch of guys to be serious about singing. To help us learn to sing with the throat open, he recommended that we pretend to have a mouthful of hot mashed potatoes. "That'll open you up!"

At the time, I was still working through my vocal metamorphosis, changing from a boy soprano to a high tenor and trying to establish some sort of equilibrium. Professor Hays took me under his wing and began to tutor me privately at no charge. We focused on explicit enunciation of consonants as a means to project tone into and out of the facial mask. One weekend, Professor Hays actually drove me from the Manhattan campus to Wichita State University so that a colleague of his could hear me sing and possibly help me extend the top of my voice range. I don't remember if anything the other instructor said made an impression on me, but Professor Hays' gesture was certainly magnanimous. I hope I had enough sense to thank him properly.

Our glee club's signature selections were "The Whiffenpoof Song" (of Yale University fame) and the Alma Mata Song for the K-State. During one rehearsal, Professor Hays asked me to sing a verse of the Alma Mater solo while the chorus hummed in the background. He liked it, and afterward, that's how we always performed the song. When my brother John enrolled at K-State in 1958, he also joined the glee club. Johnny anchored the bass section and I was with the first tenors—not bad for a family of wheat farmers!

Singing became a regular part of my life once again starting in 1969. That year, our firm completed its move to midtown. Our new offices were at 345 Park Avenue, between 51st and 52nd Streets, with a second entrance on Lexington Avenue.

The area is full of landmarks. Directly south on 51st Street are the General Electric building and St. Bartholomew's church, and the Waldorf-Astoria Hotel is one block further south. To the north of 51st Street is the Seagram building, designed by the modernist architect Mies van der Rohe.

To the east on Lexington Avenue is the Citibank building, which extends from 53rd to 54th Street, with St. Peter's Church tucked under one corner. Central Synagogue is just a block away. Two blocks to the west, on Fifth Avenue at 51st Street, is St. Patrick's Cathedral. Saks Fifth Avenue, the only store in New York that made a profit during the Great Depression is on 50th Street, directly across from the Rockefeller Center buildings.

The location was desirable for our firm and turned out to be another lucky break for me. I discovered the Turtle Bay Community Music School on 52nd Street near Second Avenue, a block and a half away. One lunch hour in the summer of 1970, I walked in and asked to use a practice room, for which the charge was 50 cents per half hour. On my way out, I asked if there was an instructor who could give me lessons—"just a few."

That's how I met Carole O'Hara, who, as it turned out, had sung the role of the mother in the NBC television production of *Amahl and the Night Visitors* several years earlier. We were kindred spirits, and "just a few" lessons turned into 25 years' worth.

Carole helped me work on placing my facial, tongue and throat muscles correctly—holding the palate up and back and holding the tongue down in order to keep the throat open— and on finding the proper place from which to *project* the tone, somewhere forward of the upper portion of the facial mask. Carole also stressed the importance of phrasing and preparation. From the beginning of each phrase, the high or low note must be accounted for; the spacing of the throat opening must be ready to accommodate every note in the phrase.

Carole used analogies to make her points. "Think of your tongue and palate as forming an oval shape, like an egg," she would say. Or, "You can't be too rich or too thin, and you can't place your voice too high in your head." She also used props.

Atop her piano, next to the music board, she placed a statuette of a frog, its mouth and throat wide open in a full-throated, "Br-r-r-r-rump." She'd point to it. "Open your mouth like that."

Perhaps most important to an aspiring singer is maintaining strong breath control from the diaphragm muscle, which requires support from the buttock and thigh muscles to control the flow of air across the vocal cords. "You have to squeeze your buttocks very hard to support your diaphragm. Pretend you're holding a dime between them," she instructed. I got the picture.

All these voice-production techniques take years to master and internalize. Certainly for me they did. But even though I was studying only part-time, I made inroads on the process. And no matter how I struggled to master the technique, I always found practice and performing to be a pleasure and a welcome relief from the rigors of my daily law practice. Many a day, I would arrive with a headache. Ten minutes into my lesson, it would have disappeared.

Throughout my years at Turtle Bay, Ms. O'Hara always organized a year-end recital for her students. Initially, I studied and performed primarily operatic arias and art songs. Then, for about five years before I developed ALS, she urged me to participate in an opera workshop. Over the years, a dozen or so students performed scenes from composers like Puccini and Mozart—particularly their respective works *La Boheme* and *The Magic Flute* and especially those scenes involving duets, trios and quartets.

I learned the music while walking the boys to school in the morning, riding the subway and sitting at my piano for the last half hour before going to bed. Instead of reading for relaxation, I memorized music, learning to pronounce the words in Italian and French and singing softly to learn to hear the pitches and intervals. One of my sons remembers being lulled to sleep listening to my late-night practicing.

Prior to joining the opera workshop, I had sung with the St. Andrews Chorale group at the Madison Avenue Presbyterian Church on 74th Street for several years. Typically, New York area church and synagogue choirs and choruses consist mostly of volunteers, people like me who love to sing and do so for the sheer enjoyment of making music, along with one or two paid singers in each voice category—soprano, alto, tenor and bass. Over the years, I became acquainted with several of these professionals, who comprise a *clique*, a relatively small community of performers and accompanists in which everyone seems to know one another.

I was singing a quartet from *La Boheme* with three of my fellow students at the Turtle Bay annual recital when my legs finally gave out as a result of ALS, and I fell down on stage. Less than six months later, I was forced to stop lessons with Carol when ALS made it impossible for me to manage the two-block and four-step walk to the school. That was a sad day for me. Fortunately, not long thereafter, Maureen was passing by our corner diner and happened to notice our upstairs neighbor sitting at a booth across from a handsome younger man. Maureen stopped in to say a quick hello and was introduced to Jim Fredericks, her vocal coach, who also lived in our neighborhood. Maureen immediately recognized an opportunity for me and, within moments, Jim had agreed to come to our apartment for coaching sessions.

Jim is an expert in religious and Broadway show music, so that became the emphasis of my study for the next four years. I sat in a chair and sang, with Jim, an expert player, at the piano. To have a focus for our coaching sessions, Jim organized concert programs that we performed in my apartment for a packed house of family and friends. Jim and I sang solos and duets, and Jim would invite one or two friends from his circle to perform as well. The atmosphere was relaxed and festive, the selections were familiar favorites, and the professional voices added an extra dimension. Each concert was designed to make me look good and, of course, I loved the attention. I especially loved singing in the company of Jim and his colleagues.

My last home concert was in the summer of 2002. By then, my breath support was starting to fail, and I found it difficult to hold myself erect in the chair for more than a few minutes. During my last song, my helper Oliver held my head upright. That was the end of my lifetime hobby.

More changes lay ahead.

TURNING POINT

Though the order of loss varies, no one with ALS escapes the inevitable and complete loss of all muscle activity. This absurd turn of events occurs over a span of just three to five years.

As the muscle atrophy progresses and breathing becomes labored, ALS patients are faced with a *Hobson's choice*: Live on in a wheelchair, assisted by a life-support ventilator, a permanent tracheostomy and a stomach feeding tube, or let the disease run its course and die of respiratory failure in a matter of days or weeks. Life with disability or no life at all? The only right choice is whatever is right for each individual ALS patient.

I faced this choice seven years after my diagnosis. I had

already been relegated to a wheelchair for four years and had lived two years longer than most patients survive when the crisis came in December 2003.

Despite my limitations, at the time Maureen and I were still traveling on occasion, and we had driven to Boston to attend an evening wedding. I had not felt well during the car drive. Although the reception dinner was right in our hotel, as evening approached I regretfully told Maureen I couldn't sit through it. She went alone, and Jose and I settled in to watch a movie on TV.

The next thing I knew, I was in a hospital room (Mass General, as I later discovered) with Maureen at my bedside.

"Bob," she said, "you certainly are a trouper!"

I tried to respond but I couldn't speak. A plastic tube was jammed down my throat, connected to a large plastic hose leading to a ventilator. So I mouthed the words, "What happened?"

Maureen told me that I'd gone into respiratory failure in the hotel room the night before. The cause was aspirated bacteria, which can develop into pneumonia within 24 hours. Since my breathing capacity had already been weakened from the progression of ALS, I had rapidly succumbed.

I remembered nothing of the events Maureen described— my lungs' failing and my lips' turning blue, my caretaker Jose's mad barefoot dash to the hotel lobby, the 911 call by a hotel security guard and the ensuing emergency treatment. According to Maureen, I was barely breathing for 10 to 15 minutes. My skin had turned ashen, but when the medics started oxygen, my color returned almost immediately.

Now, a machine was pumping air into my lungs 10 to

12 times a minute. Despite the oxygen deprivation, I had been spared any diminution of my mental faculties, and for that I was profoundly grateful.

I realized how lucky I had been that Jose had been next to me and that his quick action saved my life. But I knew I was now in a real pickle—not only confined to a wheelchair but also dependent upon a trach, a ventilator and a feeding tube. The reality of the situation was explained to me. Keeping the temporary intubation tube and ventilator in place would help me survive the pneumonia. However, ensuring my long-term survival was a vastly complicated matter.

Though an ALS victim can live a normal life span with appropriate care, that care is very complex. To go on, I would need round-the-clock attendants. They would have to be trained in the use and care of all that was required to keep me breathing and nourished—operating the ventilating, suctioning and coughing machines and dealing with the tracheostomy and stomach feeding sites. Also, those attendants would have to be ever vigilant for signs of infections, particularly pneumonia.

The prospects were daunting, but having already resigned myself to the fact that I would be permanently confined to a wheelchair, I considered it a *no-brainer* to agree to the additional assistance I would need to survive. It probably would have been harder to make the decision had I not felt so well. Despite the pneumonia, I never felt any particular pain then, nor have I to this day. The worst I have experienced is occasional fatigue and some mild throbbing in my legs.

Finally, I thought of the poster campaign in the New York subway exhorting youths to stay in school: "A Mind is a Terrible Thing to Waste," it said. To those of us with ALS, the phrase is particularly poignant. Although our extremities are wasted, our minds are not, and we see, hear and feel everything. How could I possibly choose to die, I thought, when I still have my mind? Wouldn't that, too, be a terrible waste?

By coincidence, another ALS patient, also on life-support ventilation, was in the room next to me. His family gave Maureen much encouragement as well as advice for raising the necessary funds to handle the expenses of respiratory care.

Still, when I was given the facts about the new level of dependence that would be necessary, many thoughts went through my mind: Isn't this going to be just too much for Maureen to handle? Is my life worth the burden of caretaking it will place on my family? Won't I be still more of an embarrassment to my sons in a restaurant or basketball game? And how will I be able to afford the expense of caretakers 24/7 for 365 days a year? I looked to Maureen for a cue about my decision.

Her response was unhesitating. "Do it, Bob! Don't you want to see the boys get married, meet your grandchildren, and be around for everything else the future might offer?" Through all my second thoughts and worrying, Maureen has remained steadfast in her resolve that I should keep going.

REHAB

I was in the ICU at Mass General for three weeks with Maureen at my side. The most immediate concern was that I recover from the pneumonia. The memory that stays with me most clearly, however, is how swollen my tongue and throat became from the trauma when the tube was shoved down my throat by the emergency medical responders—not that I'm complaining, given the results it produced. Still, during the four days the tube remained down my throat, I was so uncomfortable I could think of little else. For three months after the tracheostomy was performed and the tube was removed, my tongue was sore.

The tube prevented me from talking for the ten days or so, and that was especially frustrating. But once the pneumonia was under control, the tube was removed and I had a permanent tracheostomy. At first, the nurses attempted to have me talk by pressing a vibrator device against the side of my throat (the type of device used by someone who has lost his or her voice box), but that was a total failure. Finally, the doctors installed a trach insert in my windpipe with an inflatable *cuff*—a small annular (ring-shaped) tire surrounding it. The cuff is left slightly deflated so air from the ventilator can pass over the vocal cords. Once it was in place, I could talk as usual. When we could communicate normally, again, both Maureen and I cried with joy. She gave me a big hug.

The personnel at Mass General had insisted that I transfer to a rehabilitation facility for a training period of two or three weeks before going home. An interim stay in rehab is the safest way—practically speaking, the only way—to help a new ventilator patient make the transition from hospital to home. The patient and his or her family need ample time to learn how to set and maintain the ventilator equipment, to follow the protocols for the medicine and feeding routines, and to care for the *stoma*—the tracheostomy site.

For the training, I traveled by ambulance from Boston to the Helen Hayes Hospital, just north of New York City. The ride was excruciating, since for its duration I was lying on the gurney with barely any padding, and I couldn't seem to get my weight off my tailbone. To make matters worse, the ambulance driver made a wrong turn, adding another thirty minutes to the four-hour trip. At least that meant that Maureen was already there when I arrived. She was at my side when the nurse directed my gurney toward a room with a bright yellow sign on the door.

It read, "CAUTION, CONTAMINATED AREA."

Maureen was appalled. "You're not putting him in there, are you?"

"No other room is available. It shouldn't be a problem."

"My husband isn't going in there. Leave him in the hallway until something else opens up."

"He can't possibly be left in the hall," the nurse protested, but nevertheless she headed to the nurse's station to huddle with the others on duty. A few minutes later, I was rolled into another room, where I stayed thereafter.

I began to accustom myself to the daily routine that would now be essential to my life. On waking and every four hours afterward, I required a ten-minute treatment with a nebulizer, a machine that sends a mist through the trachea opening to break up mucus clumps in a patient's lungs. Next, I had to be treated with an in/ex sufflator (sometimes called a coughilator) to bring up fluid. Then, to suction away any residual fluid, a catheter had to be inserted through the trachea opening to the bottom of my lung cavities.

I quickly found that I much preferred the in/ex sufflator procedure to the catheter, which irritates the wall of the lung and sets off spasms of gagging. One of the respiratory therapists commented that he had gotten more mucus from me with the sufflator than from any other patient. (I wonder if that were an achievement for which I wanted to set records.)

Next, a physical therapist went through light stretching and range-of-motion exercises: holding each leg straight and raising it to a 50° or 60° angle for ten repetitions, rotating each foot clockwise and then counterclockwise ten times, and bending each knee toward my chest ten times. The therapist would then go through a similar routine with my arms.

Afterward, aides would help me with a sponge bath, a bath in a portable bathtub, or a shower in a rolling shower chair. The latter two procedures required a great deal of effort. Two aides transferred me onto a mechanical lift device, known as a Hoyer lift, another kept the ventilator air hose from tangling and a fourth held my head and kept water from draining into the trachea opening. And a total of four transfers were required: from the bed to the lift and from the lift to the tub or shower chair, then back again.

Then two aides dressed me in street clothes every day— an essential part of the rehabilitation process. Finally, another aide transferred me back to the Hoyer lift so I could return to a wheelchair, in which I spent an increasing amount of time over the weeks.

The pneumonia ordeal had weakened me considerably. The medical community has adopted a numerical scale to assist in evaluating the overall nutritional health of a patient. On a scale of 0 to 20, a nutrition score of 17 to 20 is considered normal or good. When I was admitted to Mass General, my nutrition score was just seven. Obviously, it was very poor. Every four hours, through my stomach feeding tube, I received liquid nourishment (285 calories, a total of 1710 per day), and three times a day I got a protein supplement. This caloric intake helped me regain my strength and return to normal nutrition levels.

During week two, I was fitted for a new wheelchair to accommodate a portable ventilator and batteries. At the same time, the hospital personnel contacted a medical supply company and made lists of the equipment I would need regularly at home.

By the third week, the speech therapy staff began to work with me, experimenting with several different manual and computer-assisted communication devices. At the time, I spoke clearly enough to operate a computer with voice-recognition software.

Medicines aren't critical to the ALS patient—nothing cures the disease—but running the machinery correctly is. For the patient to breathe comfortably, the ventilator's cycles per minute, the volume of breath and the sensitivity settings must be operated correctly. The operation of the air hoses leading from the ventilator to the tracheostomy site is also critical. There are at least eight friction-fitted connections in the hosing circuit. If any one of them becomes dislodged, no air passes through, and the alarm sounds. In order to determine quickly and methodically which part has become disconnected, the caregiver must know where each hose connection is located. The patient and caregiver must also master every detail of the battery and electrical hookups, air circuitry and connections, and medicine dosages.

Even at Helen Hayes, where a trained staff attended me, my air circuit became disconnected and was incorrectly reconnected by a nurse's aide on two occasions during my transfer from the bed to the wheelchair. The minutes that passed before a respiratory nurse was able to find the error were harrowing. In case of such an emergency, a hand-operated ambulatory air bag must always be near a respiratory patient so someone can gently squeeze the bag every two or three seconds to pump air into the patient's lungs and keep him or her comfortable while the mechanical problem is resolved.

At first, the ventilation and suctioning procedures seemed too complicated to be safely performed by caretakers at home. The rehab staff urged my family to consider sending me to a nursing-home facility. The choices were limited, however, since only three in New York accepted respiratory patients.

Fortunately, Maureen's sister Diane had come from Winnipeg to help us face the challenges that lay ahead, and for that I will be eternally grateful. The two of them made field trips to assess the care the available facilities could offer. Maureen quickly concluded that the only way I could possibly hope to enjoy a reasonable quality of life was by living at home.

Once the final decision was made, all of us—me, my caregivers Jose and Oliver, and especially Maureen— determined to learn the operation of the respiratory equipment and feeding routines. Oliver was studying for a nursing examination at the time, but Jose, Maureen and Diane came to the hospital every day and the boys visited on the weekends.

As I regained strength and learned the intricacies of the respiratory settings and all the circuitry connections in the airway between the ventilator and my trachea insert, I was able to help the respiratory and occupational therapists give instructions to Maureen and Jose, and they eagerly began to give me suctions and nebulizer treatments as the therapists looked on, made corrections and offered tips and insights. Though initially mastering the operations of the machines, hoses, filters, connections, battery hook-ups, and chargers seem to be an impenetrable jumble, in time they became familiar and even simple.

There was other information to be absorbed and recorded as we acclimated to my new situation. Diane accompanied Maureen to conferences with the Helen Hayes professional staff and kept a notebook to organize all the names, numbers and locations of suppliers of wheelchairs, hospital beds and other equipment as well as a lengthy list of specialists in neurology, gastroenterology, pulmonology and otolaryngology. Diane continually encouraged Maureen and me as we mastered the routines.

Despite the seriousness of my situation, our mood wasn't grim—no small thanks to Jose. He soon was wheeling me out of the room, up and down corridors and out to the large lobby/reception areas at Helen Hayes. One day, a nurse left her stethoscope in the room. When the cute and personable young physical therapist arrived that afternoon, Jose draped the earpieces around his neck and placed the stethoscope on my chest, as if to listen for the crackling noise that signals fluid buildup in the lungs.

"I Doctor Molina," announced Jose, who has not yet lost his Ecuadorian accent. "I checked Bob's lungs—clear today. I no hear anything."

"Yeah, right…Doctor Frankenstein! That's who you are!" the therapist replied, greatly amused.

At the end of the third week, Maureen convinced the doctors and staff at Helen Hayes that she, Jose and Oliver were fully capable of handling the equipment, and they let me go home.

It was wonderful to be wheeled back into our apartment.

After six weeks in hospital rooms, my eyes had become adjusted to seeing a palette of whites and grays. The rich, warm tones that Maureen had chosen to decorate with—yellows, golds and oranges—enveloped me and literally warmed my skin. I was home again, and I knew for certain that when my time comes, it is where I want to be.

Just two months later, on February 29, 2003, we received tragic news. Diane had drowned off the coast of Guatemala. She was chaperoning a group of University of Manitoba alumni who were observing its college-credit program for service work in underdeveloped countries. After visiting a coffee plantation, the group had gone for a swim. One of the women, standing in water only knee deep, was caught by a rip tide and swept away. When Diane, who was just a few feet away, rushed to help her, she too was carried out to sea. The women hung onto one another, bobbing up and down in the ocean water. Though a boat rescued them less than half an hour later, Diane was unconscious and could not be revived. Thanks to Diane, though, the other woman survived.

Maureen's sister spent much of her life in the service of others, and that is how she died. She should be remembered as a true American heroine.

COMMUNICATION

An ALS victim experiences disability by stages. When your legs go, you're confined to a wheelchair. Losing the use of your arms, you can't do many everyday tasks. Once your hands no longer function, you can't feed or groom yourself. When you're unable to breathe or swallow independently, you have to rely on machines for oxygen and nourishment. You lose the power of speech when your tongue and jaw stop functioning. And when your facial muscles cease to function, your face becomes frozen, forming a permanent mask.

I've heard that every disabled person longs to have one less disability. The quadriplegic wishes to be only a paraplegic; the paraplegic wishes to have one good leg; the person with a limp wishes to have the leg restored to normal. So it went with me. At each stage, as my disabilities increased, I would think, that if only I could get back to where I was six months ago or only three months ago…. If only I could use my hands. If only I could speak. If only…. If only….

Though our faces show little or no expression and our bodies are still, the victims of ALS continue to have the full powers of sight and hearing as well as a normally functioning brain.

Today, I am among a small group of relatively lucky ALS victims. I was able to breathe on my own for a full seven years after the onset of the disease, and now, six years after that, I am still able to smile and open my mouth wide enough for a toothbrush. I can still move my head from side to side, to indicate "no" or "I don't know," and I can respond in the affirmative with a slight nod or two eye blinks.

To prepare myself for the loss of use of my hands and arms, I had Lasik surgery on my eyes so I wouldn't have to rely on someone to adjust and clean my glasses.

But after three years on the ventilator, I came to a point where I could no longer breathe comfortably unless the cuff was fully inflated. While that ensured that my lungs got the full volume of air with each ventilator breath, it prevented me from speaking. Eventually my helpers would constantly have to inflate the cuff to get more air to my lungs, then deflate it so I could speak, then inflate it, and so on. That went on for several weeks until it became obvious I no longer had any options. Air to my lungs was vital, and speech was not. My voice, which had been weak, was now gone altogether. Luckily for me, that period lasted less than nine months. But, during that time, I was essentially entombed in my own body—"locked in" in the words of the narrator of *The Diving Bell and the Butterfly*, who was similarly afflicted. I was unable to express myself except with a smile, a nod or a raised eyebrow.

Today, when I am out, I can communicate with friends or family only by using a small alphabet card. The letters are broken up into five lines, each line beginning with a vowel (A,B C D; E F G H; I J K L M N; O P Q R S T; U V W X Y Z). As the lines and letters are pointed out, I either shake my head "No" or nod "Yes." This laborious process effectively rules out casual conversation.

I am, however, an avid listener, and after dinner with a friend or family, I will often email my thoughts on the subject the next day with my eye-controlled computer, which speaks as I type. By giving me back my voice and letting me communicate as fully as anyone else, this device has made my life much richer and fuller. With it, I can carry on a face-to-face conversation or send emails through the Internet.

I use the computer for at least four to six hours every day. It keeps me in touch with the whole world, in as much detail as I am able or willing to absorb. When I'm *on my computer*, I feel completely normal, for I'm doing what I've always done: listening, thinking, talking and writing. I even feel younger; after all, my thought processes haven't changed that much since high school. And since I'm either in bed or sitting in the wheelchair, I have no aching back or tired feet. There is no physical pain associated with ALS.

HOSPITAL CARE

Though there is no pain with ALS, many situations are uncomfortable, particularly if a hospitalization is required.

The intensive level of personal care required for an ALS patient who is incapable of moving his or her body is simply beyond the limits of what hospitals can offer outside of an ICU. What's more, since the disease is somewhat uncommon, some of the caretakers are not thoroughly familiar with all of the protocols and support devices. In fact, the first pulmonologist I visited at Mount Sinai Hospital had never even heard of the in/ exsufflator, which by then had become a sort of lifeline for me, clearing fluid from my lungs at least a half dozen times a day.

I thought it might be useful to share some of what my experiences have taught me in the hopes it may benefit others. Regarding hospital care in general:

Though getting IV treatments is uncomfortable, a better solution may be coming. If you need an IV, a needle must be inserted into an arterial vein. Doctors are reluctant to keep a needle in one site longer than four or five days for fear of infection, so a new one must be inserted periodically. In the case of ALS patients, cancer patients and others who may have little muscle mass to support the veins, it is hard to find an arterial vein in the arm. Moreover, the vein tends to *roll*, so it's hard to place the needle in the right spot. Not every blood technician is expert in this procedure, so they may do multiple *sticks* before one is successful, and though the pain is short-lived, the experience can be a real ordeal. For the most part, I had to just *suck it up*.

During my last hospitalization, however, an ICU technician instructed the nurse in the use of a small ultrasound device to pinpoint the elusive arterial vein. The nurse was able to direct the tip of the needle accurately and successfully on the first try. This seemed to be a new piece of equipment, and I hope its use becomes routine.

A urine catheter is not an ALS-related necessity. It is inserted solely for the convenience of hospital personnel. Aside from being uncomfortable, it is a magnet for infection. Have it removed as soon as possible.

If possible, have a private caregiver come to the hospital. Outside of the ICU, *traveling nurses* who go from hospital to hospital working three 12-hour shifts per week generally provide bedside care. The lack of continuity can be a real problem, especially for someone who is totally dependent on machines. One nurse actually inflated the cuff of my trachea so I couldn't talk, saying she had no time to listen to my requests for help. Respiratory therapists make intermittent appearances to look at the ventilator settings, make a note in the patient record (obviously for a malpractice defense should the patient have expired without anyone's noticing!), and then turn on their heels and hustle away, often without a word or a smile or even eye contact with the patient.

Some staff members seem better suited to working in a morgue. I had an unpleasant experience during the hospital stay when I was still able to speak, though somewhat inaudibly. As a young intern was working on the ventilator settings, I was trying to communicate which were the most comfortable settings. The intern was unresponsive, so my caretaker spoke up.

"He's trying to tell you what the settings should be."

"Oh," said the intern. "I've never had *one of these* speak."

My caretaker was taken aback. "*One of these?* What do you mean?"

"I've never had a patient on a respirator talk to me. I had better get the respiratory people." And with that, he left.

A private caregiver can be your advocate and is also helpful to attend to personal hygiene, swab your mouth with mouthwash, clear the feeding tube, shift your body position at least every half hour, and provide light physical therapy by moving your legs and arms through a range of motion at least once daily. Moreover, just the presence of a family member or trusted caregiver can provide a great source of comfort to the ALS patient—someone who recognizes what is meant by a raised eyebrow or a head nod (no matter how slight) or someone who has a modicum of proficiency reading lip movements. In my experience, the hospital nurses invariably turned to my family or caregiver and asked, "What is he saying?" Or "What does he want?" Without this assistance, hospital stays would be very difficult.

Stretching and massage by a physical therapist once or twice a week in the hospital (and out of it) is also beneficial if you're motionless. Physical exercise is merely tiring and does nothing to maintain muscle mass in an ALS patient, but stretching maintains flexibility in the ligaments and tendons and lessens throbbing in knees and shoulders. The massaging helps maintain skin tone and conditioning.

If you have a tracheostomy there are other issues to consider.

The trachea insert device should be replaced periodically. Though this is very basic, no nurse or doctor at either Mass General or Helen Hayes mentioned it to me. I learned about it from the medical supply technician when I arrived home, six weeks after the tracheostomy was performed. By the time I got to a knowledgeable pulmonary specialist and from there to an otolaryngologist at Mount Sinai, my trachea insert had not been changed for some four months.

When the doctor first attempted to pull it out, it wouldn't budge, and he ended up ripping it from the trachea opening. This tore the granular tissue that had encircled and tightly gripped the tube leading to my windpipe, causing profuse bleeding into my lungs.

The tracheostomy has to be performed properly. The problem, I subsequently learned, was with the way the tracheostomy had initially been performed. The procedure was carried out right in my bed in the ICU, and the doctor (presumably an intern) had simply cut a circular hole in my throat and pushed the trachea insert into it and down my windpipe. Apparently, the staff had assumed I'd be dead before the granular tissue growth would be a problem.

Over the next year, I visited Mount Sinai at several two-month intervals where they attempted to cauterize the opening in my neck with a chemical burn agent. But the tissue repeatedly grew back, and at each change of insert, there would be bleeding into my lungs, which of course required immediate suctioning.

Finally, the doctors at Mt. Sinai did the procedure as it should have been done in the first place. They brought down a piece of skin from my neck to make a kind of flap that they attached to the windpipe opening in a semi-circle. This eliminated the gap between the throat opening and the windpipe. Now my caregivers can replace the insert periodically at home without incident.

For an ALS patient with a tracheostomy who is on a life-support ventilator, viral or bacterial pneumonia is the primary foe. After the tracheostomy, I had two hospitalizations, both for pneumonia. In March 2005, the doctors did a bronchoscopy procedure, which effectively removes all infectious fluids from the lungs and bronchial passages, and I was released after a week. In the fall of 2006, I was hospitalized with a double infection, one in the lungs and another in the chest wall, which was due to a particularly resistant bacterial strain. While some strains can be successfully treated with antibiotics in pill form, the more resistant ones, which, ironically, abound in hospital operating rooms and ICU areas, can be treated only with antibiotics administered intravenously.

With pneumonia, you may need a drain as well as antibiotics. For my second bout of pneumonia, a thoracic surgeon sliced a six-inch long opening in my back and snaked a tube into the chest wall just below my rib cage to the infected area. Over the next six weeks, the drain tube was backed out, ever so slowly, permitting the tube passageway to heal from the inside out. I estimate about a gallon of blood leaked out over the course of my recovery. As the surgeon daily checked the output of blood, I was tempted to ask if he was from a family of barbers.

I was kept in the thoracic ward so my doctor could follow me along with his other patients. I was astonished to discover that by comparison to them, I was the picture of health. Virtually all were suffering from lung diseases that left them obviously exhausted after only slight movements. Several coughed incessantly. As a group they were incredibly weak, and their distress was most disheartening. Although I am on a ventilator, I have never felt anything close to the suffering exhibited by those patients.

If you have pneumonia, you're better off with a coughilator. At Helen Hayes, the respiratory therapists utilize both the coughilator and a hand-manipulated catheter that can be maneuvered with a slight twisting motion into each lung. This combination ensures that fluid is removed from both lungs each time the procedure is performed. The coughilator has one more advantage: In effect, it exercises the lung walls, expanding and contracting them as the air volume is forced in and then withdrawn.

When I was there, Mount Sinai Hospital had no coughilators. They used a deep suction catheter that is encased in a soft, flexible outer sheath that permits the catheter to be pushed in and out of the lung. While the sheathing ensures sterility, it does not allow the catheter to be twisted so as to reach each lung.

The left lung anatomically is the smaller lung and somewhat set off from the windpipe. In my case, it is also the one more susceptible to pneumonia and, consequently, liquid buildup. A hospital relying exclusively on a sheathed catheter for removal of fluid buildup in the lungs is short-changing its patients, for the sheathed catheter does not reach into the left lung. And the absence of a coughilator machine means there also is no exercise of the lungs. Based on my experiences, I would urge the medical community to reassess its care for pneumonia patients, at least for ALS patients who have no other lung impairment.

ASSISTANCE

I've been more fortunate than many ALS patients because my three sons have remained in close proximity to lend a hand when needed, and Maureen has worked tirelessly to see that my medical and personal needs are met, to handle the benefits that provide financial support for my home assistants, to provide me with a full social schedule—and to drive our wheelchair-entry van like a pro!

The additional assistance of loyal and competent caregivers has been invaluable in helping me to fare so well despite my total disability.

Though in 1998 I had been sorely disappointed by the loss of support from the administrative staff at my law firm, starting with the startling departure of my secretary, I soon found a wonderful solution.

Through a nursing care agency, I connected with Oliver Pua, then a 21-year old Filipino immigrant who had been trained as a nurse but was working in a retail store. I initially hired Oliver to help with my grooming, dressing, eating and other personal routines, but I soon found that he was capable of much more.

He quickly learned the office procedures, located law books in our library and publications on the Internet, and could write English longhand as fast as I could dictate. We worked on the computer together and sat side by side for most of the day. I would pore over the books, exhibits, transcripts and opposing briefs Oliver would hand me, and then I would dictate to him (or, occasionally, a replacement secretary) my responses, answering briefs, and letters.

For more than four years, until my retirement in 2003,

Oliver remained my factotum at the law firm—serving as nurse, attendant, paralegal assistant and part-time secretary all at once. Despite my confinement to a wheelchair, thanks to him I was able to service the firm's clients to the best of my abilities. Oliver remained with me for four more years after my retirement, until he received his U.S. nursing certification. He is now a kidney dialysis specialist.

I made two other wonderful caregiver connections about that same time. The first was Abdel Zerzif, a native of Morocco who had earned his medical degree in France. In medical school here, he was working on a specialty degree in dermatology with certification in surgery. Abdel came to my apartment each morning to lift me from my bed and into the shower, shave and dress me for work—always formally, with a tie. Then he'd lift me into the car, accompany me to the office and, finally, make the transfers from the car to the office chair. Abdel was my helper for nearly two years. Having completed his degrees, he currently practices in Greenwich, Connecticut, and we remain in contact. You will never meet a kinder soul.

Then I found Jose Molina, a former semi-professional soccer player in Ecuador and Canada. His career ended when he broke his foot badly because of a misplaced kick from an opposing player. Initially, Jose covered for Abdel for just the early morning routine and went to another patient after settling me in my office chair, but he has since become my primary caregiver. Jose is fiercely loyal and remarkably strong. His athletic training means he can easily execute my lifts without assistance. But what I appreciate most of all is his delightful sense of humor. He lightens the mood every day.

In the last couple of years, I also have been fortunate

to have the assistance of Karen Jack, a knowledgeable and especially resourceful respiratory aide. In addition to providing routine respiratory care and attending carefully to my supplies, Karen indulges me with a *spa hour* on each weekly visit. I get a thorough shampoo, manicure, pedicure, shave, and a facial—all involving a variety of soaps and lotions plus a massage.

These devoted and talented people came to the U.S. from many places—Philippines, Morocco, Trinidad, Ecuador, and Poland. Some are on the way to citizenship, Jose now has his green card, and Oliver and Abel have become citizens already. America, the melting pot, is the land of opportunity—just as it was for me.

ON CHOOSING LIFE

It has been reported that a very high percentage of persons diagnosed with ALS elect not to undergo the tracheostomy/ mechanical ventilator option, also known as *invasive life support*. As many as 90% of people say no; I have seen research that puts the number even higher, up to 97%. It's less surprising when I recall that even one of the neurologists, who treated me, strongly discouraged me from choosing the trac/ventilator option.

The more positive news from the research is that among those people, who decided to go this route, over 90% are content with their decisions and would make the same choice over again—as would I.

It helps that today's mechanical ventilators are small and easily portable, and that they make breathing so comfortable that using them quickly becomes second nature. The prospect that is no doubt most frightening—reaching the point at which

ALS prohibits not only physical movement but also the ability to speak—has been mitigated enormously by the development of the eye-controlled computer, which substitutes quite adequately for the lack of speech, as I have previously noted.

I can send email messages; I can prepare, edit, save and retrieve documents; and I can conduct research on the Internet as though I were in a library. As a result, I have been able to pursue projects that are intellectually challenging and allow me to function as a professional.

I was able to use my voice for the first three years after my recovery from the pneumonia and acclimation to speaking with the trachea insert. During that time, I helped commercialize the patents and trademarks of a mascara-application system that my niece Jenni had developed several years earlier. We were in contact almost daily, attending meetings, suggesting proposals for licensing agreements, drafting press releases and business plans for possible joint ventures or capital investment. We have been able to continue our collaboration by computer. The project is ongoing.

I continue to serve as a kind of *consigliere*—a trusted advisor—to friends and business acquaintances who call on me for my legal and technical expertise.

For one case, I reviewed a series of lengthy trust agreements. That required my studying legal treatises and case law from several states regarding the interpretation of these instruments. I prepared a detailed memorandum analyzing the trusts and drafted numerous letters that our friend might use in subsequent discussions with the various different trustees. After two years of work, the case concluded to our side's satisfaction.

As I write this, the parties are awaiting resolution on

another case in which there are three wills at issue, one including several codicils made by the testator as his health deteriorated shortly before his death. These wills are still under scrutiny by the interested heirs and others claiming entitlement to the proceeds of the estates. I spent several months studying the wills to determine the controlling provisions and conferring with the friend who had consulted me on the best course of action and the likelihood of success.

After a conversation with a business associate on clean energy sources as an alternative to coal and oil, I researched the current status and capabilities of wind, solar, hydroelectric, biofuel and nuclear fission energy and prepared a *white paper* discussing my findings in laymen's terms. I concluded that it was unrealistic ever to expect the total energy from wind, solar, hydroelectric and biofuel to account for more than 20% of the nation's energy needs; that a goal should be set to produce no more than 30% of our energy from coal and oil; and that the remaining 50% of energy must come from nuclear power plants. This paper included a review of the current status of reactor technology throughout the world. Fission energy is clean, and each plant can be run at full capacity full-time, powering factories and businesses by day and recharging battery-run cars at night for clean commuter travel. Since fossil fuel is not a sustainable energy source and is a major pollutant, this goal should be mandatory. If put into effect immediately, it should be achievable by the year 2050.

For ALS patients, I hope to make two things clear. One, a diagnosis of this disease need not be a death sentence. Patients should know they can exist with it indefinitely, and successfully, as I have done for the past 12 years. Two, life is everything. And what is it but the ability to feel, think and communicate? Thanks to today's technologies, ALS can't take any of these from you.

Postscripts

END OF AN ERA

I can't say I had a plan from childhood to *make it in New York*. I merely made the most of opportunities presented to me. Each was a building block for me personally and for my career. I was a willing participant who always endeavored to do my best, but I had no idea how high the blocks would carry me. I grew from a slight, shy farm boy into a confident man, enjoying a successful law practice and raising a family in one of the most cosmopolitan centers of the world. You never know where life will take you—or your siblings.

Georgette moved to Denver shortly after World War II and dated a Navy veteran. Around 1947, he proposed, but Georgette turned him down. Shortly thereafter, she learned he had committed suicide and left behind a note directed to her. Denver newspapers carried the story and printed the note. She felt terrible, of course, but was surprised by the role she had played. She hadn't considered their relationship sufficiently deep to have contemplated marriage.

In 1949, she married Bill Leary, who in 1956 was elected Mayor of Thornton, Colorado, a new suburb of Denver. He later was appointed a district judge for Westminster County, just north of the city. After years as a secretarial/accounting clerk for the Denver public schools, Georgette retired to raise her children: Ellen Kay and Stephen, in nearby Thornton.

During the years Georgette lived in Seattle and Denver, every December she sent Mom and us boys a large box plastered with stickers warning "Do Not Open Until Christmas!" Georgette's Christmas box was always a much-anticipated delivery. Sadly, Georgette's big heart gave out just before Christmas in 1984. She was only 63.

Ruth and Glenn eventually built a house in Fairbanks, Alaska and started a steel fabrication business in 1952. After Glenn died of liver cancer in 1968, Ruth ran the business for 30 years, until she retired for health reasons several years ago. The Greer steel fabrication business continues to flourish under the management of Ruth's sons, David and Mark, and her daughter Linda's husband, Stephen. I spoke to Ruth by phone the day before she died just two years ago. Her zest for life continues to be an inspiration to me.

Eleanor returned from Salina, where she had been working for Bell Telephone, and began crying her eyes out. That's how I learned that she had been engaged but her fiancé had gotten drunk at a New Year's Eve party and married another woman! I recall her discussing what to do with the ring. I think she gave it back. After staying for a while with Georgette, she returned to Salina.

Diagnosed with diabetes at the tender age of six, just a couple of years after the discovery of insulin, Eleanor had a constant struggle with the disease, constantly gauging her food intake and sugar level between injections of insulin and always carrying a piece of chocolate or other sweet to avoid going into shock when her sugar level fell too low. Mom watched Eleanor carefully, even when she was an adult. That was difficult for Eleanor, but she sometimes failed to recognize the change of mood that signaled that her sugar level had dropped and diabetic shock was imminent.

Not long after her broken engagement, Eleanor was again home on a visit when a new suitor came to our farm to pick her up. Well-dressed and polite, he drove a new car and obviously adored Eleanor. He was a strong, solid citizen-type guy— someone we felt would be helpful with her medical problems— and all of us hoped Eleanor would ultimately marry him. But she apparently couldn't get past his major drawback: He was extremely homely, like an Ichabod Crane. He must have sensed her lack of enthusiasm and soon stopped calling.

At some point her condition took a bad turn and Eleanor was hospitalized in Kansas City where she met and married Philip Randel, a fellow patient who had lost both his legs to the ravages of the disease. He was a very intelligent man who, when health permitted, made his living by restoring old or damaged photographs. I often observed him hunched over a large magnifying glass with a built-in bright fluorescent light, working with a variety of inks and extremely sharp pens. I recall his working on a photograph in which the subject's eye had been obliterated by a glare. Phillip's work was so expert that it was impossible to tell which eye had been drawn and which was the actual eye. Eleanor and he were married ten years when Phillip finally succumbed to diabetes.

She remarried. With Evan Carlson, a Swedish-American, she had five extremely happy years. She was near 70 when she died of complications from diabetes in 1993.

My brother Paul stayed close to home, making his living as

an auto mechanic in various small towns and helping us with the used cars we all drove. I think I appreciate his personality more in retrospect than I did then. He was a lovable puppy of a guy, happy-go-lucky and quick to find humor even in the midst of a predicament. Paul listened exclusively to *yee-haw* country music and loved square dancing. He and his wife, Emma, a country girl more serious than Paul, were less than 20 years old when they married. Soon they had two children, Darrell and JoAnn.

About 15 years later, Paul and Emma confounded us all by divorcing and then switching partners with another couple who had been their best friends. Eventually, both second marriages failed. Each married a third time, but Paul was eventually divorced and then Emma was widowed. Not long afterward, Paul drove to Oklahoma and asked Emma out for a cup of coffee. They remarried shortly and remained together until Emma died in 2007. A spark that flew into his eye while he was operating a welding torch several years ago affected Paul's eyesight, but at 82, he remains as light-hearted as ever. On a recent visit, he was wearing a pair of flat-heeled cowboy boots or *dancing shoes*, as he called them. He continues to square dance and clog in and around Bartlesville, Oklahoma, where he lives near his son.

Along with Eleanor and Paul, Johnny remained in Kansas. He continued to manage the family farm for many years after receiving his degree in business administration in 1961. But after meeting and marrying Kay Steele, whose father owned a sand, gravel and concrete company in Hutchinson, Kansas, he learned that business from his father-in-law, and then opened his own business. For some fifty years, John and Kay have run their sand and concrete operation just north of Hutchinson, where they raised their four children: Renee, Loren, Lon and Lyle. Lon carried on the Paulson name in nuclear engineering at K-State and Lyle did the same in the Varsity Glee Club. Lon lives and works in Wilmington, North Carolina, while Loren and Lyle work in the family business. Renee makes her home in nearby McPherson, Kansas.

When Arnold graduated from K-State in the spring of 1957, the Babcock and Wilcox Company in Lynchburg, Virginia recruited him to design reactor cores for nuclear reactor power systems. He was with them for more than 27 years and for three more years was a consultant for commercial nuclear power plants. During that time, he was assigned the position of Nuclear Advisor to the nuclear merchant ship N.S. Savannah. For nearly two years, he traveled the world on that ship, opening up ports to the concept of a nuclear-powered merchant fleet. Unfortunately, operating costs at that time were too high to be commercially feasible. The ship was taken out of service in 1971 and is now mothballed near Newport News, Virginia.

Arnold met Sara Lee Wilson, then a graduating student at Randolph-Macon Women's College in Lynchburg and they married in 1961. Within the next seven years, they welcomed their children: Thomas, Jennifer, Lynne, Lissa, and Glenn. Years later, they divorced. Arnold lives in Lynchburg, operating his own company PIMS, Inc., designing computer programs for investment management. Sara and her three daughters live in the New York area, and among them I have six great-nieces and great-nephews. We have had many family get-togethers throughout the years and I remain in close contact with all of them.

My mother continued to live on the farm until age 85,

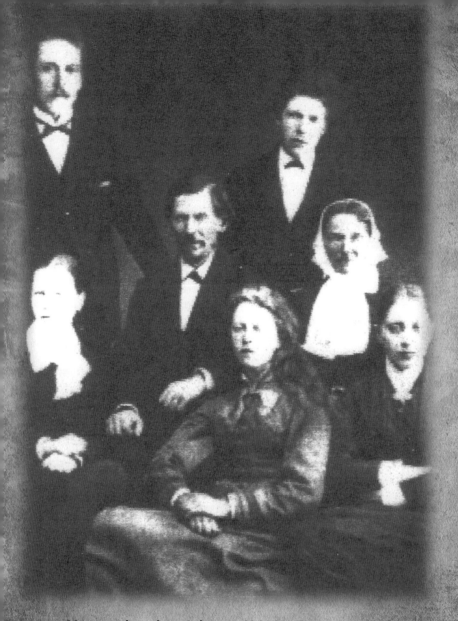

My grandmother, Johanna Kristina Petterson Karlsson
(front row center); my great-grandparents Jons
Petterson and Kjerstin Frieberg Petterson (center row);
brothers of my grandmother, Karl, August, and Swen
Petterson and grandmother's sisters, Botilda Petterson
Malmstrom and Maria Petterson (c1882)

when she suffered a stroke and was hospitalized. She died two years later. The farm was sold shortly thereafter, in 1982.

When Helga died in 1987 at age 103, the Paulson era in Lindsborg came to an end.

But events that took place in Lindsborg would have dramatic consequences for me decades afterward.

REVELATION

Just four years ago, thanks to an incredible amount of pack-ratting by my grandfather and my sister Ruth and to sleuthing by her son David Greer, I learned some startling news about my parents. The source was a postcard sent from Topeka, Kansas some ninety years before to the family farmhouse near Lindsborg.

The original home in which my grandparents had settled on our farm southeast of Lindsborg in the mid-1880's, though constructed of wood and with wood siding, was little more than a lean-to. Bit by bit, my grandfather paid off the $10,000 that the farm cost him, using the income from his crops and cattle sales.

Sometime between 1915 and 1920, the original house was rebuilt and expanded.

On May 2, 1913, a postcard from Topeka, Kansas was sent to my grandfather Jons Peter Paulson (misspelled "Poulsen") at "R.R. No. 2, Box 47, Lindsborg, Ks," signed, "Din kusin [your cousin], Thilda Malmstrom." By some quirk, that little postcard was kept in the farmhouse through its reconstruction and throughout my mother's lifetime. When Mom died in 1979, my sister Ruth took it to her home in Fairbanks, Alaska. David found it, some 90 years after it had been sent.

That little postcard holds the key to my ALS affliction.

The letter writer, "Thilda," was Bothilda Pettersson Malmstrom, the mother of cousins Ellen and Lillian, whom Mom had visited in Topeka on her way to San Francisco. Thilda had addressed my grandfather Jons Peter Paulson as "Cousin" because she and her sister Johanna Cristina Pettersson Karlsson were his first cousins. Johanna's daughter, Ellen Amalia Elisabet Karlsson, and Jons' son, Nils George Paulson, who were second cousins, fell in love. They married and had a family, and I was one of their sons.

This close mixing of bloodlines would have an unfortunate ramification—my being afflicted with ALS at age fifty-eight.

ALS is thought to be the result of a familial genetic defect in approximately 10% of all cases. Every gene in our bodies is carried in duplicate. If one of a pair is defective, the person is deemed a *carrier* but suffers no affliction. However, when two *carriers* of the same defective gene marry, there is a three in four probability—a 75% chance—that any offspring might become a carrier. What's more, the chance that any of the offspring receives a *bad* gene from both parents and might become afflicted is one in four or 25%.

The only way to snuff out these recessive genetic defects is to marry outside a common heritage. The *bad* gene will disappear within one or two generations.

Of course, if you dig back far enough into the history of mankind, we are all the product of marriages between cousins. It is estimated that no two of us are more distantly related than 50th cousins.

However, while both the Christian and Judaic religions

generally discourage marriage between first cousins, consanguinity, as it is known, is common in the Muslim countries of the Middle East such as Pakistan, Iraq and Saudi Arabia. In fact, marriage between first cousins is encouraged, particularly between a young woman and the son of her father's brother.

While there don't seem to be statistics from these countries on birth defects that may have resulted from this widespread practice, in America and Western Europe, the rate of birth defects in consanguineous marriages seems to be between four and six percent. Though this is a relatively small number, it is twice the rate that occurs in other marriages.

And in England, while Pakistanis constitute only 3% of the population, they account for one-third of that country's birth defects. That would suggest the need for careful genetic counseling to determine whether there is a potential problem if cousins who marry decide to have children.

CHROMOSOME #21

The matter of my family's genetics had come to my attention in another fashion when I was 41 and Maureen was pregnant with our second child, Luke. Maureen's gynecologist decided to run an amniocentesis test as a precautionary measure. When the initial results came back, the chromosomal studies looked suspicious, so the doctor ordered a repeat. However, because each test required three to five weeks to run, by the time the second test results came back, the pregnancy had advanced to nearly five months and the question of abortion was becoming problematic.

The second test results brought devastating news. They

seemed to positively reveal a defective #21 chromosome, which has been long known as the cause of the birth defect Down syndrome. The testing was carried out at New York's Cornell Hospital under the direction of the doctor who had personally developed the amniocentesis procedure some 25 years earlier. As an additional precaution, he recommended that Maureen and I each have our chromosomes banded—stained so they can be examined microscopically—just to be sure there was no anomaly. While we waited for the test results, the doctors and genetic specialists warned us not to expect a miracle and to make plans for dealing with a Down syndrome child.

In the meantime, the doctor gave me a printout of the chromosome bands from Luke's test and directed me to a pair of medical texts in the hospital's library that covered genetic anomalies. Sure enough, Luke's #21 chromosome was identical to the textbooks' illustrations of defective #21 chromosomes in children with Down syndrome. The evidence seemed conclusive. Meanwhile, the results on Maureen's and my chromosome banding would not be known for a week.

Emotionally shattered, we turned to Maureen's sister and her friends in Canada and to our church's pastor, John Smucker, and his wife, Irene. It was a soul-searching time as we desperately sought out specialists and clergy for information and support.

The doctor telephoned Maureen himself with the results of the tests on Maureen and me. Incredibly, my #21 chromosome was identical to Luke's. The doctor was dumbfounded. In 25 years of practice, he had seen only one other case of a normal adult with a defective #21 chromosome, an adult female in France. But I and, it seems, each of my three sons all carry a strange-looking #21 chromosome with no ill effects. Hallelujah!

EPILOGUE

Today, with the help of my caretakers and family, I continue to maintain quite a full life.

I use my ventilator to keep me going, and the in/ex sufflator first thing in the morning, usually at least twice more during the day, and the last thing at night before going to sleep. Once it removes the fluid that is building up in my lungs, usually accompanied by a brief episode of uncontrollable gagging, I breathe comfortably for the next two or three hours, or until there is another buildup, in which case the routine must be repeated.

I take no medicine specifically meant to alleviate the ALS disease because none is available. Though Riluzole has been thought to stave off death, it is effective for less than six months, so is of little use. Recently, lithium has been shown to have some effect on slowing the progression of the muscle deterioration but, for me, it is too little, too late.

So I take only small daily dosages of a mood-elevating drug to combat depression, amitriptylene to decrease saliva production in the mouth (since I no longer can swallow), and, at night, a muscle relaxant and a sleep-inducing drug that together effectively ensure a full night's sleep.

To my surprise, I have found one can do quite well without using one's legs, and the eye-controlled computer and mechanical ventilator very capably substitute for my incapacity to breathe, speak and write on my own. What cannot be replaced, however, and what I miss a great deal, is the ability to manage my arms and hands and the chance to eat and drink. But in exchange for a fully functioning brain and my eyesight, it is a small price to pay.

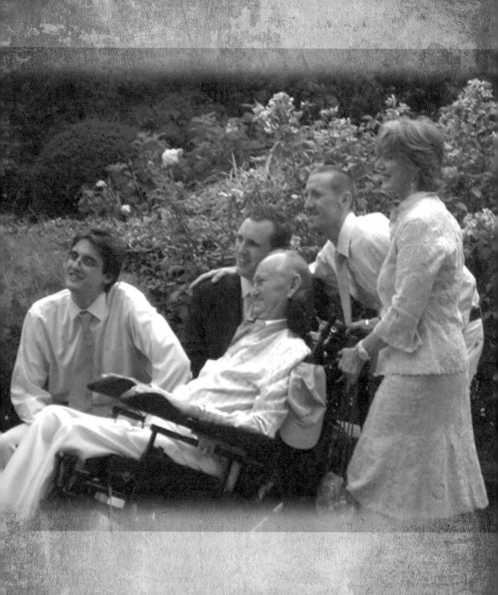

My family, from left,
Jake, Joshua, Luke
and Maureen (2007)

There are also psychological issues associated with ALS to confront and overcome—or at least accept, if only with resignation. Total dependence on caregivers for every physical movement means a certain loss of control that is often frustrating and sometimes exasperating. And no matter how well a task is done, as we all know, if someone else does it, it's never 100 percent right.

At first, confinement to a wheelchair makes one incredibly self conscious to the point of embarrassment. Conversation at a stand-up affair is virtually impossible except for those willing to lean over within hearing range. The wheelchair occupant constantly wonders if strangers looking his way feel pity or sympathy. Either way, it's an assault to one's ego. Then there are the instances when people don't bother even to look at the person in the wheelchair, treating the occupant as a non-entity, and instead, speaking only to the attendant. That is a particularly galling indignity to endure. Over time, however, these moments of embarrassments have faded—in particular since the time I have been able to communicate with my computer. The fact that I can no longer control drooling or spasmodic gagging engenders still further embarrassment in a public setting. I have spent a lifetime educating myself intellectually and socially, developing sufficient savoir-faire to be comfortable in a variety of social settings—and now, I can no longer just meld into the crowd. As my son Josh once put it, when my party and I enter any room, "We cut a rather wide swath." My wheelchair will forever be the first thing that people notice about me, but I hope it is not the thing that defines me.

As I reflect on my life's journey, it seems I have been the recipient of a string of good fortunes that followed some sort of plan. It was as if step-by-step I was prepared for what lay ahead.

My childhood experiences performing vocal, instrumental and piano music helped make me comfortable in a public setting. My mother's determination and my own ongoing efforts to make a living on the farm gave me an appreciation and understanding of what it takes to compete and persevere. My stint on the college debating team was invaluable training for my later career in law. My early exposure to farm machinery and tools, as well as my formal education in engineering, prepared me for interacting with inventors and grasping a variety of technical subject matter. My early life taught me to use a practical, common-sense approach for solving the daily problems we faced on the farm. In law school, this common-sense approach proved invaluable grounding for my development of a sense of good judgment in resolving legal and factual issues.

But I also see that something in me always drove me forward, fueling my desire to reach goal after ever-higher goal. Perhaps then, I made some of my own good luck.

In any event, I am at peace—satisfied with my choices, knowing I did all that I could with the skills I was given, and grateful to my parents, who gave me life; my brothers and sisters, who give me a helping hand; and my family, who've given me reason to be proud and their love. I am a lucky man.